Living
the ■
g.i.
diet

DELICIOUS RECIPES
AND REAL-LIFE STRATEGIES
TO LOSE WEIGHT
AND KEEP IT OFF

RICK GALLOP
AND
EMILY RICHARDS

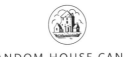

RANDOM HOUSE CANADA

www.randomhouse.ca

National Library of Canada Cataloguing in Publication

Gallop, Rick
    Living the G.I. diet : delicious recipes and real-life strategies to
    lose weight and keep it off / Rick Gallop, Emily Richards.

Includes index.
ISBN 0-679-31253-6

1. Glycemic index. 2. Reducing diets—Recipes. I. Richards, Emily II.
Title. III. Title: Living the glycemic index diet.

RM222.2.G343 2003   613.2'5   C2003-903053-9

Printed in Canada

10 9 8 7 6 5

For the thousands of readers who have shared their stories and successes with me and who gave me the inspiration and motivation to write this book

Contents

Introduction

In 2002, I launched my first book, *The G.I. Diet,* with some trepidation. It wasn't the diet's effectiveness that I was worried about—far from it. I knew from personal experience that it was the best weight-loss program available. The book was based on the latest scientific research and had been endorsed by a number of physicians. I myself had lost twenty pounds on it after all but giving up hope of ever slimming down. What did concern me was that it might get lost in the sea of diet books crowding bookstore shelves—books that were full of empty promises, that promoted diets that were dangerously unhealthy or that simply did not work.

I wanted to let people know the real cause of their weight problem and that they could lose the extra pounds easily, without having to perform difficult mathematical calculations or having to go hungry. I'm convinced that the reason Canadians are gaining more weight than ever before is because they have simply been given the wrong information. The truth is you can eat as much or even more than you currently do and still slim down. All you have to do is choose the right foods.

Fortunately, people took notice of *The G.I. Diet* and it clearly hit a chord with them. The book became a national bestseller, and tens of thousands of Canadians have lost weight on the program! It is so rewarding to receive everyone's e-mails describing their successes—and they are the real motivation behind my writing this second book, *Living the G.I. Diet*. I wanted to provide even more information and lots of wonderful recipes to help you continue losing pounds or to maintain your new weight.

For those of you who didn't read *The G.I. Diet*, I've started this book with a short outline of its principles. This summary will give you everything you need to get started on the program right away. If you feel, however, that you need a more detailed explanation, you may want to read my first book. Those of you who are already familiar with the program can read the summary for a quick refresher or just skip over it. I should mention, though, that the G.I. Diet Food Guide on page 20 has been expanded to include even more foods than appeared in the first book.

I've also decided to enlist the help of experts in writing this book. I've asked my wife, Dr. Ruth Gallop, to write a chapter on how to deal with the emotional reasons why we eat. She is a professor at the University of Toronto and an international authority on childhood trauma and its impact on our behaviour as adults. Though not all of us have suffered trauma, most of us do use food for reasons other than physiological need. If you have a bad day at work, do you buy a box of chocolates on your way home? If you're alone on a Saturday night, do you indulge in a tub of Häagen-Dazs ice cream? Ruth will tell you how to ease

Dear Rick,

I tried several diet plans throughout the last thirty years. . . . None of them worked for any length of time. And all the weight I lost came back threefold.

I was riding my exercise bike and watching the news when the health segment came on. They talked about *The G.I. Diet* and raved about the results some people had had with it. Best of all, they talked about the fact that the diet would lower cholesterol, and keep your sugar levels low. This sounded good to me, as my family has a history of diabetes, and I was a very good candidate to develop this disease in the next few years.

So I went out and purchased the book and began to read it that night. I couldn't put it down! It all made perfect sense and was written in a way that was easily understood, and best of all: NO MEASURING ANY FOOD!

I have lost a total of 63 pounds, and have dropped from a size 28 (which was a very tight 28) to a size 18! More important than the weight loss is the fact that my last blood work done by my doctor was unbelievable. My cholesterol levels have dropped dramatically and I am now in the normal levels–a big change from almost having to go on medication to control it! I feel that the G.I. Diet is the best! The world would not be in such dire straits with the obesity problems if everyone went G.I.

Thanks for listening.

Pamela

yourself out of the habit of turning to food for comfort when you are feeling stressed or depressed.

I've also asked Emily Richards, who you may know as the co-host of the popular TV show *Canadian Living Cooks,* to create a cornucopia of delicious green- and yellow-light recipes for breakfast, lunch, snacks, dinner and yes, even dessert. You can eat a wide variety of flavourful, appealing dishes on this program and never feel as though you are on a diet. In fact, many of them are sure to become family favourites.

To further motivate you, I've shared some of the e-mails I've received from people who are on the G.I. Diet. Their stories are often moving and truly inspiring. I am so proud of them and so grateful for their feedback. I hope that their experiences will help you as you embark on your journey to a new, slim you!

PART ONE

The G.I. Diet in a Nutshell

CHAPTER ONE

The Secret to Easy, Permanent Weight Loss

For years doctors, nutritionists and government officials have told us that the way to maintain a healthy weight is to eat a low-fat, high-carbohydrate diet. So if you've ever tried to lose weight, you've probably started by reducing the amount of fat that you eat. Instead of having bacon and eggs for breakfast, you switched to cornflakes with skim milk. Instead of eating a hamburger at lunch, you opted for chicken noodle soup and a slice of white bread without butter. Instead of snacking on potato chips, you munched on a couple of rice cakes. You made these healthier choices, felt good about yourself, and at the end of the month, you eagerly weighed yourself again—to find that you'd gained another two pounds! What happened?

Well, first of all, let's dispel a widely held myth: fat does not necessarily make you fat. Fat consumption in this country has remained virtually constant over the past ten years, while obesity numbers have rocketed. Obviously fat isn't the culprit. But that doesn't mean you can eat all the fatty foods you want. Most fats can be quite harmful to your health. It's alarming to read some of the popular diet books on the market today and find that they advocate eating lots of cream, cheese and steak. These foods are all high in saturated fat, which can thicken arteries, leading to heart attack and stroke. There is also increasing evidence that colon and prostate cancer as well as Alzheimer's are associated with high levels of saturated fats. These are definitely the "bad" fats and are easily recognizable because they solidify at room temperature and almost always come from animal sources. There are two exceptions to this rule: coconut oil and palm oil are two vegetable oils that are also saturated. Because these oils are cheap, they are used in many snack foods, especially cookies.

There are three other types of fat: the "best," the "acceptable," and the "really ugly." The "really ugly" fats are potentially the most dangerous. They are vegetable oils that have been heat-treated to make them thicken. These hydrogenated oils or trans fatty acids take on the worst characteristics of saturated fats. So don't use them and avoid foods whose labels list hydrogenated oils or partially hydrogenated oils among their ingredients. Many crackers, cereals, baked goods and fast foods contain these really ugly fats, but since labelling of nutritional components has until just recently been voluntary in Canada (unlike in the United States), you'll find that some packages do not list their ingredients. A good rule of thumb is to avoid these foods,

COOKING OILS/FATS

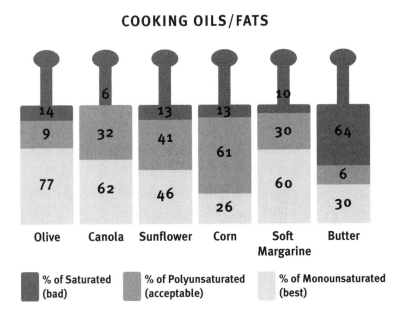

				10	
14	6	13	13		
9	32	41		30	64
			61		
77	62	46		60	6
			26		30
Olive	Canola	Sunflower	Corn	Soft Margarine	Butter

■ % of Saturated (bad)   ▨ % of Polyunsaturated (acceptable)   ▫ % of Monounsaturated (best)

because the manufacturer probably has something to hide.

So we're avoiding the "bad" fats and the "really ugly" fats, but we mustn't eliminate fat entirely from our diet. Fats are absolutely essential to our health as they contain various key elements that are crucial to the digestive process. The "best" fats are monounsaturated fats and they are found in foods like olives, peanuts, almonds and olive and canola oils. Monounsaturated fats actually have a beneficial effect on cholesterol and are good for your heart. So try to incorporate them into your diet and look for them on food labels. Most manufacturers who use them will say so, because they know it's a key selling point for informed consumers.

Another highly beneficial oil, which is in a category of its own, contains a wonderful ingredient called omega-3. This oil is found in coldwater fish such as salmon and in flax and canola seeds, and it's extremely good for your heart health. "Acceptable" fats are the polyunsaturated fats because they are cholesterol free. Most vegetable oils, such as corn and sunflower, fall into this category.

By now you must be wondering what causes people to gain weight if it isn't fat. Well, the answer lies in something you've probably never thought of as fattening at all—and that's grain. Have you noticed the multiplying number of grocery store shelves dedicated to products made from flour, corn and rice? Supermarkets now have huge cracker, cookie and snack food sections; whole aisles of cereals; numerous shelves of pastas and noodles; and baskets and baskets of bagels, rolls, muffins and loaves of bread. In 1970 the average North American ate about 135 pounds of grain. By 2000 that figure had risen to nearly 200 pounds! This staggering increase helps explain why nearly half of Canadian adults are overweight, and why 1 in 7 are considered obese—that's a 24 percent increase over the past five years! We're definitely eating too much grain, but the other half of the problem is the *type* of grain we're eating, which is generally highly processed. Take flour, for instance. Today's high-speed flour mills use steel rollers rather than traditional grinding stones to produce an extraordinarily finely ground product. The whole wheat is steamed and scarified by tiny razor-sharp blades to remove the bran and the endosperm. Then the wheat germ and oil are removed because they turn rancid too quickly to last on supermarket shelves. What's left after all that processing is then bleached and marketed as all-purpose flour. This is what almost all the breads, bagels, muffins, cookies, crackers, cereals and

GRAIN CONSUMPTION (pounds per capita)

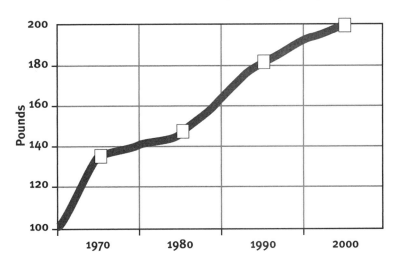

Source: U.S. Department of Agriculture

pastas we consume are made of. Even many "brown" breads are simply artificially coloured white bread.

And it's not just flour that's highly processed nowadays. A hundred years ago most of the food people ate came straight from the farm to the dinner table. Lack of refrigeration and scant knowledge of food chemistry meant that most food remained in its original state. However, advances in science, along with the migration of many women out of the kitchen and into the workforce, led to a revolution in prepared foods. Everything became geared to speed and simplicity of preparation. We now have instant rice and potatoes, as well as entire meals that are ready to eat after just a few minutes in the microwave.

The trouble with all this is that the more a food is processed beyond its natural state, the less processing your body has to do to digest it. And the quicker you digest your food, the sooner you are hungry again and the more you tend to eat. We all know the difference between eating a bowl of old-fashioned, slow-cooking oatmeal and a bowl of sugary cold cereal. The oatmeal stays with you—it "sticks to your ribs" as my mother used to say—whereas you are looking for your next meal only an hour after eating the bowl of sugary cereal. Our fundamental problem, then, is that we are eating foods that are digested by our bodies too easily. Clearly we can't wind back the clock to simpler times, but we need to somehow slow down the digestive process so we feel hungry less often. How can we do that? Well, we have to eat foods that are *slow-release,* that break down at a *slow and steady rate* in our digestive system, leaving us feeling fuller for longer.

There are two clues to identifying slow-release foods. The first is the amount of fibre in the food. Fibre, in simple terms, provides low-calorie filler. It does double duty, in fact, by literally filling up your stomach so that you feel satiated; and by taking much longer to break down in your body, so the digestive process is slowed and the food stays with you longer. There are two forms of fibre: soluble and insoluble. Soluble fibre is found in foods like oatmeal, beans, barley and citrus fruits, and has been shown to lower blood cholesterol levels. Insoluble fibre is important for normal bowel function and is typically found in whole wheat breads and cereals and most vegetables.

The second tool in identifying slow-release foods is the glycemic index, or G.I., which is the basis of the G.I. Diet and the secret to successful weight management. It was developed by Dr. David Jenkins, a professor of nutrition at the University of Toronto. Early in his career, he became interested in diabetes, a disease that hampers the body's ability to process carbohydrates and sugar (glucose). Sugar therefore stays in the bloodstream instead of going into the body's cells, resulting in hyperglycemia and potentially coma. At the time Dr. Jenkins was beginning his research, carbohydrates were severely restricted in a diabetic's diet because they quickly boost the sugar level in the blood stream. But because the primary role of carbohydrates is to provide the body with energy, diabetics were having to make up the lack of calories through a high-fat diet, which provides energy without boosting sugar levels. Now doctors were in a real quandary: although they were saving diabetics from hyperglycemia, they were accelerating their risk of heart disease.

Dr. Jenkins wondered if all carbohydrates are the same. Are some digested more quickly and as a result raise blood sugar levels faster than others? And are others slow-release, resulting in only a marginal increase in blood sugar? The answer, he discovered, is yes. In 1980, he published an index—the glycemic index—showing the various rates at which carbohydrates break down and release glucose into the bloodstream. The faster the food breaks down, the higher the rating on the index, which sets sugar at 100 and scores all other foods against that number. The chart on the next page contains some examples of G.I. ratings.

By eating only those foods that have a low G.I. rating, diabetics were now able to keep their glucose levels low and avoid hyperglycemia.

Sugar	100	Rice (basmati)	58	Apple	38
Baguette	95	Muffin (bran)	56	Yogurt (low fat)	33
Rice	87	Potatoes (new/boiled)	56	Fettuccine	32
Cornflakes	84	Popcorn (light)	55	Beans	31
Potatoes (baked)	84	Orange	44	Grapefruit	25
Donut	76	All-Bran	43	Yogurt (no fat/no sugar)	14
Cheerios	75	Oatmeal	42		
Bagel	72	Spaghetti	41		
Raisins	64	Tomato	38		

As it turns out, the G.I. also has exciting implications for anyone who wishes to lose weight. It has been proven that keeping glucose levels low is the key to permanent weight loss. This is how it works: When you eat a high-G.I. food, your body rapidly converts it into glucose. The glucose dissolves in your bloodstream and spikes its glucose level, giving you that "sugar high." The chart on page 15 illustrates the impact of digesting sugar on the level of glucose in your bloodstream compared with kidney beans, which have a low G.I. rating.

As you can see, there is a dramatic difference between the two. What is also apparent from the chart is that after your glucose level spikes, it quickly disappears from your bloodstream, leaving you feeling starved of energy and looking for more fuel. Something most of us experience regularly is the feeling of lethargy that follows an hour or so after a fast-food lunch, which generally consists of high-G.I. foods. The surge of glucose followed by the rapid drain leaves us feeling sluggish and hungry. So what do we do? Around mid-afternoon we look for a quick sugar fix, or snack, to bring us out of the slump. A few cookies or a bag of chips—also high-G.I.

G.I. IMPACT ON SUGAR LEVELS

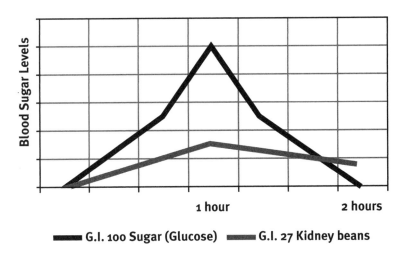

■■■ G.I. 100 Sugar (Glucose) ■■■ G.I. 27 Kidney beans

foods—cause another rush of glucose, which again disappears a short time later. And so the vicious cycle continues. Eating a diet of high-G.I. foods will obviously make you feel hungry more often and you will end up eating more as a result. Low-G.I. foods, on the other hand, are the tortoise to the high-G.I. foods' hare. They break down in your digestive system at a slow, steady rate. Tortoise-like, they stay the course, making you feel full longer, and consequently, you eat less.

There is a second reason why you should avoid eating high-G.I. foods when you are trying to lose weight. When you experience a rapid spike in your blood sugar, your pancreas releases the hormone insulin. Insulin does two things extremely well. First, it reduces the level of glucose in your bloodstream by diverting it into various body tissues for immediate short-term use or by storing it as fat—which is why glucose disappears so quickly. Second, it inhibits the conversion of body fat back into glucose for the body to burn. This evo-

Dear Rick,

I am thrilled with my 50-pound weight loss (in less than four months) and the significant reduction in my blood sugar. Your book has given me renewed hope in getting my weight off, as I have 50 more pounds to go. It is so confidence-building to know that it is not my fault for my morbid obesity these past many years, and I only wish I had known this information years ago. I cannot thank you enough!

Irene

lutionary feature is a throwback to the days when our ancestors were hunter-gatherers, habitually experiencing times of feast or famine. When food was in abundance, the body stored its surplus as fat to tide it over the days when there wouldn't be much to eat. Insulin was the champion in this process, both helping to accumulate fat and then guarding its depletion.

Today, everything has changed but our stomachs. We don't have to hunt for food anymore—there's a guaranteed supply at the supermarket. But our insulin continues to store fat and keep it intact. As everyone knows, our bodies must be able to access and draw down from our fat cells in order to lose weight. To allow that to happen, you need to do two things. First, you must consume fewer calories than your body needs in order to burn up those fat stores. Now, I hate to bring up calories since we've probably all been driven nearly over the edge with having to count them and perform complex mathematical calculations with them. But unfortunately, unless one denies the basic laws of thermodynamics, the equation never changes: consume more calories than you expend and the surplus is stored in the body as fat. That's the inescapable fact. Few diet books today mention calories, but they're there, hidden behind the various rules and suggestions. Don't worry, though, because with *Living the G.I. Diet* you can easily reduce your calorie intake without having to do any calculations and without going hungry—I'll explain how in a moment.

The second thing we must do to enable our bodies to use up its fat cells, is to keep our insulin levels low, which means avoiding high-G.I. foods. Remember the cornflakes, chicken noodle soup, white bread and rice cakes that were mentioned at the beginning of this chapter? Well, you would never lose weight if you ate those foods on a daily basis because they all have high G.I. ratings—they raise your insulin levels to the point where your body won't burn up those fat stores. Instead, you should stick to low-G.I. foods. Instead of having cornflakes for breakfast, have porridge or homemade muesli. Instead of lunching on chicken noodle soup, enjoy a bowl of homemade lentil soup. Avoid the rice cakes when you need a snack, and have a handful of hazelnuts or almonds instead. It isn't difficult to substitute low-G.I. foods for high-G.I. ones, but by making these changes, your weight will begin to drop. It's that easy. How will you know which foods are high-G.I. and which ones are low? In the next chapter you'll find a comprehensive chart that identifies the foods that will make you fat and those that will allow you to lose weight. Don't expect the foods in the latter category to be limited and boring—there are so many tasty and satisfying choices that you won't even feel as though you are on a diet. And later in this book, Emily Richards will give you many delicious ways to prepare them.

Dear Rick,

I lost over forty pounds in just over two months (from 210 pounds to 170 pounds). No more headaches! My blood pressure is back down from 180/120 to a normal reading— my doctor can't believe the change. This is the best I've felt in years. I weigh less than I did the day I got married sixteen years ago. I'm not hungry between meals with your meal plans and yes, I can indulge once in a while without putting any weight back on.

Many, many thanks,

Joe

CHAPTER TWO

The G.I. Diet

Now that you understand the science behind the G.I. Diet, it's time to get down to the nitty gritty. Basically, you need to know what, when and how much to eat to start shedding those extra pounds. Let's begin by addressing the "what." As you know from the last chapter, the key to losing weight is to eat foods that have two essential characteristics: a low calorie content and a low G.I. rating. To help you identify those foods, I have developed an easy-to-use reference tool called the G.I. Diet Food Guide.

The G.I. Diet Food Guide

This chart lists every food you can think of in one of three categories based on the colours of a traffic light. Foods listed in the red-light or "stop" category are high-G.I., high-calorie foods that should be avoided. Some of these may surprise you, for example, melba toast, mashed potatoes, turnip and watermelon are all red-light. Your body digests them so quickly that you are hungry again an hour later. Foods in the yellow-light or "caution" category—for example, sourdough bread, corn and bananas—have moderate G.I. ratings, but they do raise insulin levels to the point where weight loss is not going to happen. Foods in the green-light or "go ahead" category are the ones that will allow you to lose weight. Chicken, long-grain rice and asparagus are all green-light foods. Eat them and watch your weight drop. After you've had a chance to look over the G.I. Diet Food Guide, we'll talk about how to make it work for you.

The G.I. Diet Food Guide

BEANS	RED	YELLOW	GREEN
	Baked beans with pork		All beans (canned or dried)
	Broad		Baked beans (low fat)
	Refried beans		Black-eyed peas
			Chickpeas
			Soybeans
			Split peas

BEVERAGES	RED	YELLOW	GREEN
	Alcoholic drinks*	Diet soft drinks (caffeinated)	Bottled water
	Fruit drinks	Milk (1%)	Club soda
	Milk (whole or 2%)	Red wine*	Decaffeinated coffee (with skim milk, no sugar)
	Regular coffee	Regular coffee (with skim milk, no sugar)	Diet soft drinks (no caffeine)
	Regular soft drinks	Unsweetened fruit juices	Light instant chocolate
	Sweetened juice		Milk (skim)
			Tea (with skim milk, no sugar)

* In Phase II a glass of wine and the occasional beer may be included.

BREADS	RED	YELLOW	GREEN
	Bagels	Pita (whole wheat)	100% stone-ground whole wheat*
	Baguette/ Croissants	Whole grain breads	Homemade muffins (see p. 240)
	Cake/Cookies		Homemade pancakes (see pp. 119 and 121)
	Cereal/Granola bars		Whole grain, high-fibre breads (2½ to 3 g of fibre per slice)*
	Corn bread		
	Doughnuts		
	English muffins		
	Hamburger buns		
	Hot dog buns		
	Kaiser rolls		
	Melba toast		
	Muffins		
	Pancakes/Waffles		
	Pizza		
	Stuffing		
	Tortillas		
	White bread		
CEREALS	**RED**	**YELLOW**	**GREEN**
	All cold cereals except those listed as yellow- or green-light	Shredded Wheat Bran	All-Bran
			Bran Buds
			Fibre First
	Granola		Homemade Muesli (p.115)
	Grits		Kashi Go Lean
	Muesli (commercial)		Oat bran
			Porridge (large-flake oatmeal)
			Red River

* **Use a single slice only per serving.**

CEREAL GRAINS	RED	YELLOW	GREEN
	Couscous	Corn	Barley
	Croutons		Buckwheat
	Millet		Bulgur
	Rice (short grain, white, instant)		Quinoa
	Rice cakes		Rice (basmati, wild, brown, long grain)
			Wheat berries

CONDIMENTS/ SEASONINGS	RED	YELLOW	GREEN
	Ketchup		Garlic
	Mayonnaise		Herbs/Spices
	Tartar sauce		Hummus
			Mayonnaise (fat free)
			Mustard
			Soy sauce (low sodium)
			Teriyaki sauce
			Vinegar
			Worcestershire sauce

DAIRY	RED	YELLOW	GREEN
	Cheese	Cheese (low fat)	Buttermilk
	Chocolate milk	Cream cheese (light)	Cheese (fat free)
	Cottage cheese (whole or 2%)	Ice cream (low fat)	Cottage cheese (1% or fat free)
	Cream	Milk (1%)	Fruit yogurt (fat and sugar free)
	Cream cheese		
	Ice cream	Frozen yogurt (low fat, low sugar)	Ice cream (low fat and no added sugar, e.g., Breyers Premium Fat Free, Nestle's Legend No Added Sugar)
	Milk (whole or 2%)	Sour cream (light)	
	Sour cream	Yogurt (low fat)	
	Yogurt (whole or 2%)		Milk (skim)

FATS AND OILS	RED	YELLOW	GREEN
	Butter	Corn oil	Almonds*
	Coconut oil	Mayonnaise (light)	Canola oil*/seed
	Hard margarine	Most nuts	Flax seed
	Lard	Peanut oil	Hazelnuts*
	Mayonnaise	Salad dressings (light)	Macadamia nuts*
	Palm oil	Sesame oil	Mayonnaise (fat free)
	Peanut butter (all varieties)	Soft margarine (non-hydrogenated)	Olive oil*
	Salad dressings (regular)	Sunflower oil	Salad dressings (fat free)
	Tropical oils	Vegetable oils	Soft margarine (non-hydrogenated, light)*
	Vegetable shortening		
			Vegetable oil sprays

FRUITS	RED	YELLOW	GREEN
FRESH	Cantaloupe	Apricots (fresh)	Apples
	Dates	Bananas	Blackberries
	Honeydew melon	Kiwi	Blueberries
	Watermelon	Mangoes	Cherries
		Papaya	Grapefruit
		Pineapple	Grapes
			Lemons
			Oranges (all varieties)
			Peaches/Plums
			Pears
			Raspberries
			Strawberries

* Limit quantity (see serving size on p. 28).

FRUITS	RED	YELLOW	GREEN
BOTTLED, CANNED, FROZEN, DRIED	All canned fruit in syrup	Dried apricots	Applesauce (without sugar)
	Applesauce containing sugar	Dried cranberries	Frozen berries
	Most dried fruit*	Fruit cocktail in juice	Mandarin oranges
			Peaches in juice or water
			Pears in juice or water

FRUIT JUICES**	RED	YELLOW	GREEN
	Fruit drinks	Apple (unsweetened)	
	Prune	Cranberry (unsweetened)	
	Sweetened juices	Grapefruit (unsweetened)	
	Watermelon	Orange (unsweetened)	
		Pear (unsweetened)	
		Pineapple (unsweetened)	

MEAT, POULTRY, FISH, EGGS AND SOY	RED	YELLOW	GREEN
	Ground beef (more than 10% fat)	Ground beef (lean)	All seafood, fresh, frozen or canned***
	Hamburgers	Lamb (lean cuts)	Back bacon
	Hot dogs	Pork (lean cuts)	Beef (lean cuts)
	Processed meats	Turkey bacon	Chicken breast (skinless)
	Regular bacon	Whole omega-3 eggs	Ground beef (extra lean)

* For baking, it is okay to use a modest amount of dried fruit.
** Always eat the fruit rather than drink its juice.
*** Avoid breaded or battered seafood.

RED	YELLOW	GREEN
Sausages		Lean deli ham
Sushi (it's the rice)		Low-cholesterol liquid eggs (Break Free/Omega Pro)
Whole regular eggs		
		Sashimi
		Soy/whey protein powder
		Tofu
		Turkey breast (skinless)
		Veal

PASTA*	RED	YELLOW	GREEN
	All canned pastas		Capellini
	Gnocchi		Fettuccine
	Macaroni and cheese		Macaroni
	Noodles (canned or instant)		Penne
	Pasta filled with with cheese or meat		Spaghetti/Linguine
			Vermicelli

PASTA SAUCES	RED	YELLOW	GREEN
	Alfredo	Sauces with vegetables (no added sugar)	Light sauces with vegetables (no added sugar)
	Sauces with added meat or cheese		
	Sauces with added sugar or sucrose		

SNACKS	RED	YELLOW	GREEN
	Bagels	Bananas	Almonds**
	Bread	Dark chocolate (70% cocoa)**	Applesauce (unsweetened)

* Try to use whole wheat or protein-enriched pasta. Limit quantity (see serving size on p. 28).
** Limit quantity (see serving size on p. 28).

Candy	Ice cream (low fat)	Canned peaches/pears in juice or water
Cookies	Most nuts*	Cottage cheese (1% or fat free)
Crackers	Popcorn (light, microwaveable)	Food bars (see p. 258)
Doughnuts		Fruit yogurt (fat and sugar free)
French fries		
Ice cream		Hazelnuts*
Jell-O (all varieties)		Homemade muffins (p. 240)
Muffins (commercial)		Ice cream (low fat and no added sugar, e.g., Breyers Premium Fat Free, Nestle's Legend No Added Sugar)
Popcorn (regular)		
Potato chips/ Pretzels		
Raisins		Most fresh fruit
Rice cakes		Most fresh vegetables
Sorbets		Soy nuts*
Tortilla chips		
Trail mix		

SOUPS	RED	YELLOW	GREEN
	All cream-based soups	Canned chicken noodle	All homemade soups made with green-light ingredients
	Canned black bean	Canned lentil	Chunky bean and vegetable canned soups (e.g., Healthy Request, Healthy Choice, Too Good To Be True)
	Canned green pea	Canned tomato	
	Canned split pea		
	Puréed vegetable		

SUGAR & SWEETENERS**	RED	YELLOW	GREEN
	Corn syrup	Fructose	Aspartame
	Glucose		Equal
	Honey		Splenda

* Limit quantity (see serving sizes on p. 28).
** See sweeteners on pp. 261–62.

Molasses		Stevia	
Sugar (all types)		Sugar Twin	
		Sweet'N Low	

VEGETABLES RED	YELLOW	GREEN	
Broad beans	Artichokes	Arugula	Lettuce (all varieties)
		Asparagus	
French fries	Beets	Avocado*	Mushrooms
Hash browns	Corn	Beans (green/wax)	Olives*
Parsnips	Potatoes (boiled)	Bell peppers	Onions
Potatoes (instant)	Pumpkin	Broccoli	Peas
		Brussels sprouts	Peppers (hot)
Potatoes (mashed or baked)	Squash	Cabbage	Pickles
Rutabaga	Sweet potatoes	Carrots	Potatoes (boiled new)*
Turnip	Yams	Cauliflower	Radishes
		Celery	Snow peas
		Collard greens	Spinach
		Cucumbers	Swiss chard
		Eggplant	Tomatoes
		Kale	Zucchini
		Leeks	

* Limit quantity.

Servings and Portions

The G.I. Diet Food Guide makes choosing the right foods for your new eating plan easy. But how much of them should you eat and when? First of all, this isn't a deprivation diet. For the most part, you can have as much of the green-light foods as you like. There are only a few exceptions, which have a higher G.I. rating or calorie content than others. I've listed them along with their recommended serving sizes below.

Green-light breads (which have at least 2½ to 3 grams of fibre per slice)	1 slice
Green-light cereals	½ cup
Green-light nuts	8 to 10
Margarine (non-hydrogenated, light)	2 teaspoons
Meat, fish, poultry	4 ounces (about the size of a pack of cards)
Olive/canola oil	1 teaspoon
Olives	4 to 5
Pasta	¾ cup cooked
Potatoes (boiled new)	2 to 3
Rice (basmati, brown, long grain)	⅔ cup cooked
PHASE II	
Chocolate (70% cocoa)	2 squares
Red wine	1 5-ounce glass

Some readers have asked me if it's okay to eat twelve apples a day or an entire tub of cottage cheese at a sitting! I don't recommend that you go overboard on quantities of anything. Moderation is key. It's also important that you spread your daily calorie intake evenly throughout the day. If your digestive system is busy processing food and steadily supplying energy to your brain, you won't be looking for high-calorie snacks. I know that many people make a habit of skipping breakfast in the morning, but this is a big mistake. People who miss breakfast leave their stomachs empty from dinner to lunch the next day, often more than sixteen hours! No wonder they overeat at lunch and then look for a sugar fix mid-afternoon as they run out of steam. Always eat three meals—breakfast, lunch and dinner—as well as three snacks—one mid-morning, one mid-afternoon and one before bed—each day. And try to consume approximately the same amount of calories at each principal meal. If you eat a tiny breakfast and then a tiny lunch, you'll feel so hungry by dinner time that you won't be able to stop yourself from overeating.

As well, each meal should contain some vegetables or fruit, some protein and some type of whole grain food. Fruits, vegetables and grains are all carbohydrates, which are the primary source of energy for your body. They are rich in fibre, vitamins and minerals, including antioxidants, which we now believe play a critical role in protecting against disease—especially heart disease and cancer. That's one of the reasons why high-protein diets, which unfortunately have become quite popular in recent years, are so harmful to your long-term health. They prescribe eating a great deal of animal protein, which is high in saturated fat, while severely cutting back on carbohydrates. This causes ketosis, a dangerous electrolyte imbalance and an acid build-up in the blood that can lead to kidney damage, kidney stones and osteoporosis. Side effects include fatigue, headache, nausea, dizziness and bad breath. By minimizing the amount of vegetables, fruits, whole grains and legumes you consume, you deprive your body of essential vitamins and minerals.

With that in mind, vegetables and fruit, most of which are low-calorie and low-G.I., form the base of the G.I. Diet. Now, I know that Canada's Food Guide to Healthy Eating suggests that grains should be the largest component of your diet, followed by vegetables and fruit. But by giving grains priority, the guide is promoting the leading cause of overweight and obesity. Recently, the Mayo Clinic, one of the world's leading medical research centres, has begun to promote vegetables and fruits as the basis of a healthy diet, rather than grains, and Health Canada has decided to review its guidelines.

Protein is another essential part of your diet. One-half of your dry body weight is made up of protein, i.e., your muscles, organs, skin and hair, and protein is required to build and repair body tissue. It is also much more effective than carbohydrates or fat in satisfying hunger. It acts as a brake in the digestive process and will make you feel fuller longer as well as more alert. So please include some protein in every single meal. Too often we grab a hasty breakfast of coffee and toast—a protein-free meal. Lunch is sometimes not much better: a bowl of pasta with a few slivers of chicken. And a typical afternoon snack of a cookie, piece of fruit or muffin contains not a gram of protein. Generally, it's not until dinner that we eat protein, usually our entire daily recommended allowance plus some extra. But because protein is a critical brain food, providing amino acids for the neurotransmitters that relay

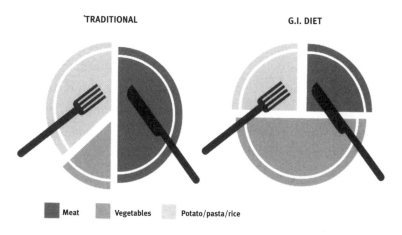

TRADITIONAL G.I. DIET

Meat   Vegetables   Potato/pasta/rice

messages in the brain, it would be better to load up on it earlier in the day. That would give you an alert and active mind for your daily activities. The best solution, however, as I've said, is to spread your protein consumption throughout the day to keep you on the ball and feeling full. Choose low-fat proteins such as lean or low-fat meats that have been trimmed of any visible fat; skinless poultry; fresh, frozen or canned fish (but not the kind that's coated in batter, which is invariably high in fat); shellfish; beans; low-fat dairy products like skim milk (believe it or not, after a couple of weeks of drinking it, it tastes just like 2%), low-fat yogurt without sugar, and low-fat cottage cheese; low-cholesterol liquid eggs; and tofu.

An easy way to visualize the portion sizes you should be consuming is to imagine your plate divided into three sections. Half the plate should be covered with vegetables and fruit. One of the sources of protein listed above should occupy one quarter of the plate, and the last quarter should be filled with a green-light type of rice, pasta or potato. Above is a diagram of what your green-light dinner plate should look like.

What to Have for Breakfast

My favourite breakfast of all time is good old-fashioned oatmeal. Not only is it low-G.I. and low-calorie, but it also lowers cholesterol. Be sure to use the large-flake variety and not the one-minute or instant oats, which have been processed. Oatmeal will stay with you all morning and it is easy to prepare, especially in the microwave. You can also endlessly vary the flavour by adding non-fat, sugar-free, fruit-flavoured yogurt; unsweetened applesauce, or fruit. Emily has included some fabulous breakfast ideas, starting on page 113. To make your regular breakfasts green-light, here are some general guidelines to follow.

Coffee

The principal problem with coffee is its caffeine content. There is growing evidence to suggest that caffeine causes your body to produce high levels of insulin—which is the last thing we want. That's why I recommend you drink only decaffeinated coffee when you are trying to lose weight. If you simply can't face the day without a cup of java, caffeine intact, then please, go ahead and have it. But don't add sugar—use a sugar substitute instead—and add only 1% or skim milk. I have received so many e-mails from readers who feel that caffeine deprivation is a definite deal breaker. If you follow the other principles of the G.I. Diet, you can have your morning cup of coffee and still reach your weight-loss target.

Juice/Fruit

Always eat the fruit rather than drink its juice. Juice is a processed product that is more rapidly digested than the parent fruit. To illustrate the point, diabetics who run into an insulin crisis and are in a state of hypoglycemia (low blood sugar) are usually given orange juice because it's the fastest way to get glucose into the bloodstream. A glass of juice has 2½ times the calories of a fresh whole orange.

Cereals

Aside from porridge, go for the high-fibre products that have at least 10 grams of fibre per serving. Oat bran is also excellent. Though these cereals are not much fun in themselves, you can liven them up with fresh or canned fruit, nuts, and non-fat, sugar-free, fruit-flavoured yogurt. You can also add sweetener (though stay away from sugar).

Toast

Always use bread that has at least 2½ to 3 grams of fibre per slice. Most of the nutrient content labels on breads list fibre for a two-slice serving, which should be 5 to 6 grams. Remember, however, that a green-light serving is only *one slice* per meal. A good choice of bread is 100% stone-ground whole wheat. "Stone-ground" means the flour has been ground with stones rather than steel rollers, resulting in a coarser grind and a lower G.I. rating.

Spreads

Do not use butter. The latest premium brands of non-hydrogenated soft margarine are acceptable and the light versions even more so, but still use them sparingly. In fruit spreads, look for the "extra fruit/sugar-reduced" versions. These taste terrific and are remarkably low in calories.

Dear Rick,

Like many others, I'm sure, I've tried different approaches to losing weight and eating healthier, but I still find myself engaged in the same battle, month after month. I used to blame it on age. I'm getting older, getting bigger, losing the hair on my head just to watch it grow on my back—now that's a pretty picture. I'd better stop. After reading your book, I understand and feel better about a whole lot of things.

Thank God for me because I love oatmeal and eat it every morning. . . . I believe, therefore I'm doing it. I eat better, I exercise more and it won't be long before I lose the remaining eleven pounds. I recently went home for Mother's Day. My sister-in-law said, "Dan, I find it so funny that before, you would eat like a bird, and now you say you are following a diet, but you haven't stopped eating." She was right and it is funny because I am losing weight and I feel great. I'm going to my grandmother's this weekend. I'm sure she'll get a good laugh when I walk in with my bag of oatmeal.

Thanks, you've made a difference.

Dan

Loblaws's Too Good To Be True brand is a particularly good buy.

Eggs

By far the best option is whole eggs in liquid form (e.g., Break Free and Omega Pro), which you can buy in cartons in the egg and dairy section of your grocery store. Because the fat and cholesterol levels have been reduced, liquid eggs are great green-light products. Use them to whip up delicious omelettes.

Bacon

Sorry, but regular bacon is a red-light food. Acceptable alternatives are Canadian back bacon, turkey bacon and lean ham.

Dairy

Low-fat dairy products are a great source of protein in the morning. I always have a glass of skim milk with breakfast. Try moving down from 2% to 1% to skim in stages. I find that 2% tastes like cream now!

Low- or non-fat yogurts that do not contain sugar, and 1% or fat-free cottage cheese and cream cheese are also excellent sources of protein. Try to stay away from other cheeses, though, since they are generally high in saturated fat.

What to Have for Lunch

Since most of us spend the lunch hour away from home, either at work or school, we tend to have two options for the midday meal: (1) we can brown bag it, or (2) we can eat at a restaurant. In both cases, eating the green-light way is definitely doable—but there are some important guidelines to keep in mind.

Brown-Bagging It

This is really the best option for the G.I. dieter. When you pack your own lunch, you can be sure that all the ingredients used are green-light. Here are some tips for turning your brown-bag into a green-light bag.

Sandwiches

This popular lunchtime mainstay is usually high-G.I. and high-calorie. But there are several things you can do to make your sandwich green-light. First, use one slice of 100% stone-ground whole wheat or other high-fibre bread. Spread on some mustard or hummus (no butter or margarine) and top with 4 ounces of lean deli ham, chicken, turkey or fish. Add at least three vegetables, such as lettuce, tomato, cucumber or green pepper. And do not top the sandwich with another slice of bread, simply eat it open-faced. Avoid egg- and tuna-salad sandwiches that are made with fattening mayonnaise.

Salads

Salads are almost always green-light but are often short on protein. Add in chickpeas or other types of beans, tuna, salmon, tofu or 4 ounces of skinless, cooked chicken breast or other lean meat. Also watch the dressing. Use only low-fat or fat-free versions. There are some great salad recipes starting on page 143.

Soups

In general, commercially canned soups have a relatively high G.I. rating because of the necessary high temperatures used in the canning process. There are a few green-light brands, such as Campbell's Healthy Request, Healthy Choice and Too Good To Be True. Homemade soups made with green-light ingredients are the best option, and Emily has provided some recipes starting on page 129. Beware of all cream-based or puréed vegetable soups, since they are high in fat and heavily processed.

Pasta

The thing to watch out for here is quantity. Your pasta dish should contain only ¾ cup of cooked, whole wheat pasta, as well as 1 cup of vegetables, ¼ cup of light pasta sauce, and 4 ounces of chicken or lean deli meat.

Cottage Cheese and Fruit

A fast and easy lunch to take to work is cottage cheese and fruit. Pack 1 cup of 1% cottage cheese and 1 cup of green-light fruit.

Dessert

Always have some fresh fruit for dessert. Pass on other sweet things at lunch time.

Lunching Out

I have provided a handy removable page of tips for eating out at restaurants on page 269. Basically, all you have to do is order an entrée that includes a low-fat source of protein, such as chicken or fish, and vegetables. Ask for extra vegetables in lieu of potatoes or rice, since restaurants tend to serve the red-light versions. Eating at a fast-food outlet, however, is another story. Because fast food is loaded with saturated fat and calories, with rarely a gram of fibre in sight, it is usually a good idea to avoid it. It's true that some major fast-food chains have recently started offering lower-fat options, but by going into the restaurant, you are walking into a den of temptation, surrounded by people scarfing down their usual fare of dietary disasters. If your alternatives are limited, however, here are some guidelines for navigating this gastronomic minefield.

Burgers

Dispose of the top of the bun and don't order cheese or bacon. Keep it as simple as possible.

Fries

DON'T. A medium order of McDonald's fries contains 17 grams of fat (mostly saturated), about 50 percent of your total daily allowance.

Milkshakes

DON'T. The saturated fat and calorie levels are unbelievable.

Wraps

An increasingly popular alternative to the traditional sandwich is a wrap. Request a whole wheat pita if available and ask that it be split in half.

Submarines

One fast-food chain that should be applauded is Subway Subs. Its entire product range is low fat. An open-faced whole wheat sub is the basis of a reasonable green-light meal. Avoid cheese and mayonnaise unless they're low fat.

Fish or shellfish

Both are excellent choices providing there's no batter or breaded coating.

Chinese

My best advice is to steer clear of Chinese restaurants when trying to lose weight. The rice is a problem, because it is usually the high-G.I., glutinous kind that tends to stick together. The sauces, especially the sweet and sour ones, are high in sugar and the noodles are also high G.I.

What to Snack On

I can't stress enough how important it is to have three snacks every day. Snacks play a critical role between meals by giving you a boost when you most need it. Choose fruit; non-fat, sugar-free yogurt; 1% cottage cheese; raw vegetables, nuts, and Emily's snack recipes on pages 233 to 245. Watch out for other products that claim to be fat- and sugar-free, such as pudding. Unfortunately these products are usually made with highly processed grain and are red-light. An exception is the ready-to-eat, soy-based pudding from President's Choice—it is green-light and tastes delicious. You might also want to look into food bars. Choose 50- to 65-gram bars that have around 200 calories each with 20 to 30 grams of carbohydrates, 12 to 15 grams of protein and 5 grams of fat. Balance and Power Protein bars are a good choice, and Shoppers Drug Mart's own brand is a best buy. The rest are often high-G.I., high-calorie, and contain lots of quick-fix carbs. Check labels carefully.

What to Have for Dinner

The typical North American dinner comprises three things: meat or fish; potato, pasta or rice; and vegetables. Together, these foods provide an assortment of carbohydrates, proteins and fats, along with other minerals and vitamins essential to our health.

Meat/Fish

Most meats contain saturated fat, so it's important to buy lean cuts and trim off all the visible fat. Chicken and turkey are excellent choices *provided all the skin is removed.* And fish and shellfish (not breaded) are also wonderful. In terms of quantity, the best measure for meat or fish is your palm. The portion should fit into the palm of your hand and be about as thick. Another good visual is a pack of cards.

Potatoes

The G.I. ratings of potatoes vary from high to moderate, depending on how they are cooked. Boiled new potatoes are the only kind you should eat, two or three at a sitting. Baked, mashed and fried potatoes are all red-light.

Pasta

Though most pastas have a moderate G.I. rating and are low in fat, they have become a villain in weight control. That's because we tend to eat too much of it. Italians quite rightly view pasta as an appetizer or side dish, while North Americans make it a main course with sauce and a few slivers of meat. Pasta should only make up a quarter of your meal (about ¾ cup cooked). Use whole wheat or protein-enriched pasta and stay away from cream-based sauces.

Rice

Rice also has a broad G.I. range. The low ones are basmati, wild, brown and long-grain because they contain a starch, amylose, that breaks down more slowly than that of other rices. Serving size is critical, too. Allow 50 grams of dry rice or ⅔ cup cooked per serving.

Vegetables/Salad

Eat green-light vegetables and salad to your heart's content. Serve two or three varieties of vegetables at every dinner as well as a salad.

Desserts

There is a broad range of low-G.I., low-calorie desserts that taste great and are good for you. Virtually any fruit qualifies and there's always low-fat, sugar-free ice cream. And wait till you try Emily's Baked Chocolate Mousse (page 251) and Pecan Brownies (page 254)!

Beverages

We all know that we are supposed to drink eight glasses of fluids per day. Personally, I find this a bit steep. But I do try to drink a glass of water before each meal and snack. Other than to stay hydrated, I do this for two reasons: one, having your stomach partly filled with liquid before the meal means you will feel full more quickly, thus reducing the temptation to overeat; two, you won't be tempted to wash down your food before it's been sufficiently chewed.

Water is definitely the best beverage choice because it doesn't contain any calories. Liquids don't seem to trip our satiety mechanisms, so it's a waste, really, to take in calories through them. Alcohol especially is a disaster for weight control because it is easily metabolized by the body, resulting in increased insulin production—so try to avoid it. It is also wise to stay away from fruit and vegetable juices, which we digest rapidly. If water is too boring for you, there are a number of no-cal or low-cal beverages to choose from.

Coffee

If you can, it's best to stick with decaffeinated coffee (see page 32). Never add sugar and use only 1% or skim milk.

Tea

Both black and green teas have considerably less caffeine than coffee and also contain antioxidants that are beneficial to your heart health. Two cups of tea have the same amount of antioxidants as seven cups of orange juice or twenty of apple juice! So tea in moderation is fine, but use a sugar substitute if you normally add sugar, and 1% or skim milk. Herbal teas are also a good choice, though they do not contain the antioxidants that black and green teas have.

Soft Drinks

Most soft drinks are high in both sugar and caffeine, and are therefore red-light. Instead, opt for diet soft drinks that do not contain caffeine.

Skim Milk

Personally, my favourite beverage is skim milk. It's non-fat, and since most lunches tend to be a bit protein deficient, drinking skim milk is a good way of making up for some of the shortfall.

Soy Milk

Soy milk can be an excellent choice, but buyer beware: most soy beverages are not only high in fat, but also have added sugar. Look for soy milk that is non-fat or low-fat, that has no flavouring like vanilla or chocolate and that has no added sugar.

Vegetarians

If you are a non-meat eater and need to lose weight, the G.I. Diet is the program for you. All you have to do is continue to substitute vegetable protein for animal protein—something you've been doing all along. However, because most vegetable protein sources, such as beans, are encased in fibre, your digestive system may not be getting the maximum protein benefit. So try to add some easily digestible protein boosters like tofu and soy protein powder to your meals.

Okay, you now know what, when and how much to eat and drink to start shedding those pounds! In the next chapter, I'll outline the steps for getting started on the G.I. Diet.

CHAPTER THREE

Getting Started in Phase I

The G.I. Diet consists of two phases, and the first, Phase I, is really the most exciting. This is the weight-loss portion of the diet, when you're putting your newly acquired knowledge into practice, developing healthier eating habits, trying new recipes, watching your waistline diminish and feeling more energized. Once you have achieved your weight-loss goal, you enter Phase II—a heady moment. At this point all you have to do is maintain your new svelte frame, and perhaps buy some new clothes. Ready? Here are the essential first steps for launching yourself into Phase I.

Step 1: Set the Goal

Before you do anything else, get your vital statistics on record. I can't think of a greater motivator than measuring your progress as the pounds drop off. On page 273, you will find a detachable log sheet to keep in the bathroom and record your weekly progress. Always weigh yourself at the same time of day, because a meal or bowel movement can throw off your weight by a couple of pounds. First thing in the morning, before you eat breakfast, is a good time. Another measurement that is important to know is your waist circumference. It indicates your level of abdominal fat, which is significant to your health, especially your heart health. A woman's health is at risk if her waist circumference is 32 inches or more, and a man's is at risk if his is 37 inches or more. A measurement of 35 inches plus for women and 40 inches plus for men puts you in the high-risk category for heart attack and stroke. People with a high level of abdominal fat, whom doctors describe as apple-shaped, have a much higher chance of developing cardiovascular disease and Type 2 diabetes.

To measure your waist, take a measuring tape and wrap it around your natural waistline just above the navel. Don't be tempted to suck your stomach in! Just stand in a relaxed position and keep the measuring tape from cutting into your flesh. Now record your weight and waist measurement on the log sheet. I've added a Comments column so that you can also note how you're feeling, or any unusual events in the past week that might have some bearing on your progress. (Readers have asked for additional log sheets. I suggest you photocopy some extra copies before you start.)

Now that you know what your current weight and waist measurement are, you should set your weight-loss target. How much do you want to lose? The best method for determining this is the Body Mass Index, or BMI. It is the only internationally recognized standard for measuring body fat—which is the only part of you that we're interested in reducing. The BMI table on pages 48 to 49 is very simple to use. Just find your height in the left vertical column and go across the table until you reach your current weight, or the closest number to it. At the top of that column is your BMI, which is a pretty accurate estimate of the proportion of body fat you're carrying—unless you are under 5'0", are elderly or overly muscled (and you really have to be a dedicated bodybuilder to qualify). If any of these characteristics apply to you, then these numbers, in all probability, do not.

The ideal BMI is between 20 and 25. This range is quite generous, however, and your target BMI should be toward the lower end, preferably around 22. BMI values under 18.5 are considered underweight, while those between 25.0 and 29.0 are classified as overweight. BMI values of 30.0 and over are considered obese. So put your finger on the BMI number 22 in the chart and drop down until you reach your height, which is shown in the left margin. The number at that intersection is what your weight should be to achieve that BMI target. Let's look at an example. If Sharon is 5'6" and weighs 161 pounds, her BMI is 26, which is 4 notches above her target BMI of 22. This means that Sharon has to lose 24 pounds in order to bring her to her 22 BMI goal of 136 pounds.

Generally it will take between three and six months to achieve your BMI target. How do I figure that? Well, a pound of fat contains around 3,600 calories. To lose that pound in one week, you must reduce your caloric intake by around 500 calories per day (500 x 7 = 3,500 calories). So if you want to lose twenty pounds, it will take twenty weeks. If that seems like a long time to you, think of it in terms of the rest

BODY MASS

BMI	NORMAL						OVERWEIGHT						OBESE
	19	**20**	**21**	**22**	**23**	**24**	**25**	**26**	**27**	**28**	**29**	**30**	**31**
HEIGHT	WEIGHT (POUNDS)												
4'10"	91	96	100	105	110	115	119	124	129	134	138	143	148
4'11"	94	99	104	109	114	119	124	128	133	138	143	148	153
5'0"	97	102	107	112	118	123	128	133	138	143	148	153	158
5'1"	100	106	111	116	122	127	132	137	143	148	153	158	164
5'2"	104	109	115	120	126	131	136	142	147	153	158	164	169
5'3"	107	113	118	124	130	135	141	146	152	158	163	169	175
5'4"	110	116	122	128	134	140	145	151	157	163	169	174	180
5'5"	114	120	126	132	138	144	150	156	162	168	174	180	186
5'6"	118	124	130	136	142	148	155	161	167	173	179	186	192
5'7"	121	127	134	140	146	153	159	166	172	178	185	191	198
5'8"	125	131	138	144	151	158	164	171	177	184	190	197	203
5'9"	128	135	142	149	155	162	169	176	182	189	196	203	209
5'10"	132	139	146	153	160	167	174	181	188	195	202	209	216
5'11"	136	143	150	157	165	172	179	186	193	200	208	215	222
6'0"	140	147	154	162	169	177	184	191	199	206	213	221	228
6'1"	144	151	159	166	174	182	189	197	204	212	219	227	235
6'2"	148	155	163	171	179	186	194	202	210	218	225	233	241
6'3"	152	160	168	176	184	192	200	208	216	224	232	240	248
6'4"	156	164	172	180	189	197	205	213	221	230	238	246	254

Source: U.S. National Heart, Lung and Blood Institute

INDEX (BMI)

		OBESE						EXTREME OBESITY					
32	33	34	35	36	37	38	39	40	41	42	43	44	45
WEIGHT (POUNDS)													
153	158	162	167	172	177	181	186	191	196	201	205	210	215
158	163	168	173	178	183	188	193	198	203	208	212	217	222
163	168	174	179	184	189	194	199	204	209	215	220	225	230
169	174	180	185	190	195	201	206	211	217	222	227	232	238
175	180	186	191	196	202	207	213	218	224	229	235	240	246
180	186	191	197	203	208	214	220	225	231	237	242	248	254
186	192	197	204	209	215	221	227	232	238	244	250	256	262
192	198	204	210	216	222	228	234	240	246	252	258	264	270
198	204	210	216	223	229	235	241	247	253	260	266	272	278
204	211	217	223	230	236	242	249	255	261	268	274	280	287
210	216	223	230	236	243	249	256	262	269	276	282	289	295
216	223	230	236	243	250	257	263	270	277	284	291	297	304
222	229	236	243	250	257	264	271	278	285	292	299	306	313
229	236	243	250	257	265	272	279	286	293	301	308	315	322
235	242	250	258	265	272	279	287	294	302	309	316	324	331
242	250	257	265	272	280	288	295	302	310	318	325	333	340
249	256	264	272	280	287	295	303	311	319	326	334	342	350
256	264	272	279	287	295	303	311	319	327	335	343	351	359
263	271	279	287	295	304	312	320	328	336	344	353	361	369

of your life. What's less than half a year compared with the many, many years you'll spend afterwards with a slim, healthy body? This isn't a fad diet—fad diets don't work. The G.I. Diet is a wholesome, realistic, surefire route to permanent weight loss, and you can do it! Let's move on to step 2.

Step 2: Clear Out the Cupboards

At this point, your kitchen cupboard and refrigerator still probably contain some of the foods that are listed in the red-light column of the G.I. Diet Food Guide. Now how are you going to reach your goal with all this temptation at your fingertips? Give yourself a break and do something radical: clear out your pantry, fridge and freezer of all red- and yellow-light products. If the thought of throwing them in the garbage makes you blanch, donate the canned foods and other non-perishables to the local food bank and give the rest to neighbours, your children away at college or anyone you know who doesn't happen to live in your house. This does not mean you will be depriving the non-dieters in your family—this is a healthy way of eating for everyone. You're doing them a service!

Step 3: Go Shopping

After you've enjoyed a good meal—and you're not remotely hungry—head over to the local grocery store and stock up on green-light foods. Before you go, you might also want to turn to Emily Richards's recipe section later in this book and pick out some new dishes to try. To make your first green-light shopping excursion simpler, I've included a detachable grocery list on page 267, which you can take with you. On it, you will find dried apricots listed—though they are yellow-light, they can be used in Emily's recipes.

I've tried to include a broad range of products in the G.I. Diet Food Guide, but of course I couldn't hope to include all the thousands of brands available in most supermarkets. Check labels when in doubt, and look for three things in particular: 1. Check the calorie content per serving and that the serving size is realistic. Some manufacturers will low-ball the serving size in order to make the calories or fat content appear lower than that of their competitors' products. 2. Check the fat content, especially of saturated fat or trans fatty acids (usually called hydrogenated), and look for a minimum ratio of 3 grams of poly- or mono-unsaturated fat to each gram of saturated fat. The total amount of fat should be less than 10 grams per serving. 3. Note the fibre content, since fibrous foods have a lower G.I. rating. Look for a minimum of 4 to 5 grams of fibre per serving. You will probably be buying more fruit and vegetables than usual, so be a little daring and try some varieties that are new to you.

Step 4: Start Eating the Green-Light Way

Altering one's eating habits always requires some additional thought and preparation initially. As you begin to eat the green-light way, you will most likely have to consult the G.I. Diet Food Guide often. Before long, however, choosing the right foods will become second nature. To make starting the new plan as easy as possible, I suggest that you choose one or two standard breakfasts that you can eat every day for the first couple of weeks. This may sound boring, but you most likely do this now without thinking much about it. Perhaps you always have a bowl of cornflakes with fruit, or a toasted bagel with cream cheese. Decide what you are now going to have and give yourself enough time each morning to prepare and eat it. I myself look forward to starting each day with a bowl of oatmeal. I vary its flavour by adding different types of fruit yogurt or sliced fruit or berries. You'll find more breakfast ideas on pages 113 to 127.

While your dinner preparation routine is unlikely to change, lunches and snacks, because they are often eaten away from home, will require some extra forethought. As I said earlier, you can eat the green-light way at restaurants, but the best option is to brown bag it. Make any of the soups in the recipe section of this book ahead of time and store them in lunch-size quantities in the freezer. You could also prepare one of Emily's salads the night before. Another suggestion would be to make extra when you are preparing dinner and have the leftovers for lunch the next day.

Be sure to plan out your snacks as well. Keep adequate supplies of ready-to-eat snacks such as fruit yogurt, cottage cheese, nutrition bars, fruit and nuts at home, at work, in your purse, in your briefcase and in the car. Bake other green-light snacks, such as Emily's Cranberry Cinnamon Bran Muffins, ahead of time and store them in the freezer. You can allow them to thaw in your lunch bag or defrost them in the microwave. A little preparation will ensure that you'll always have the right foods on hand when those inevitable hunger pangs strike and will go a long way in guaranteeing your success on this diet.

Dear Rick,

I have Type 2 diabetes, hypertension and I'm over 100 pounds overweight. My husband had recently been tested for high cholesterol and needed to lose 25 pounds or so. We emptied our fridge and pantry over a period of time and, armed with your excellent shopping guide, bought most of what we thought we'd need for the first week of the diet. I made up three pages of quick-reference breakfast, lunch, supper and snack ideas and taped them up in the kitchen.

We started eating right exactly eight weeks ago. My husband has lost 20 pounds and is waiting for the results of his cholesterol test. I have lost fourteen pounds and a few inches around my waist. But the most remarkable thing is that my sugar levels have normalized. . . . My doctor says if things continue this way, I may be able to go off insulin completely. During my checkup last week we discovered that my blood pressure was normal for the first time in years.

This is the first time that I have not felt hungry while trying to lose weight. There have been MANY challenges but your hints, especially about eating out, have made it so much easier. I keep apples, yogurt and almonds at my two places of work and a Balance Bar and glucose tablets in my purse in case I miss a snack between jobs or if I get too busy.

I have turned at least ten people on to your marvellous book and all of them are losing weight and feeling great. Thank you for making it relatively easy for a lot of desperate people to quietly try something and succeed.

Yours sincerely,

Margie

Step 5: Add Some Exercise to Your Routine

Dieting has a far greater impact on weight loss than exercise does. To give you some idea of how much exercise is required to lose just one pound of weight, have a look at the table below.

	EFFORT REQUIRED TO LOSE 1 LB OF FAT	
	130-lb person	160-lb person
Walking (4 mph–brisk)	53 miles/85 km	42 miles/67 km
Running (8 min/mile)	36 miles/58 km	29 miles/46 km
Cycling (12–14 mph)	96 miles/154 km	79 miles/127 km
Sex (moderate effort)	79 times	64 times

Clearly, an exercise regimen alone is not enough to reach your weight-loss goal, even if you are a sexual athlete! However, exercise is an important factor in *maintaining* your desired weight. For example, if you were to walk briskly for a half hour every day for one year, you would burn up calories equalling twenty pounds of fat. Exercise increases your metabolism—the rate at which you burn up calories—even after you've finished exercising! As well, it builds muscle mass, and the larger your muscles, the more energy (calories) they use. So start walking, bicycling, lifting weights, doing resistance exercises or playing sports. Not only will it help your weight-loss efforts, it will dramatically reduce your risk of heart disease, stroke, diabetes and osteoporosis.

These five steps will get you well on your way to achieving your weight-loss target. Don't be surprised if you lose more than one pound per week during the first few weeks as your body adjusts to the new plan. Most of that initial weight will be water, not fat—remember, 70 percent of your body weight is water. Please don't worry if from time to time you "fall off the wagon." I probably live about 90 percent within the program and 10 percent outside it. It's important that you don't feel as though you're living in a straitjacket. The fact is that I feel better and more energized when I stick to green-light foods, and you will too. Try to keep your lapses to a minimum—they will marginally delay your target date. Once you have reached your goal, you will be able to allow yourself more leeway in Phase II.

CHAPTER FOUR

Phase II

When you're ready to begin Phase II of the G.I. Diet, hearty congratulations are in order: you've reached your weight-loss target! You stuck to the principles of the program and are looking and feeling great as a result. All you have to do now is maintain your new weight. While this is definitely a less onerous phase than the first, maintenance can also be a challenge. In fact, those of you who have lost weight in the past only to regain it soon after may find the thought of Phase II a daunting prospect. I recently received an e-mail from a reader who lost forty-three pounds in just six months on the G.I. Diet. Though she had reached her ideal BMI of twenty-two, she was terrified of moving into Phase II in case she gained the weight back. Statistics tell us that 95 percent of people who lose weight on a diet tend to put it back on. However, before you start feeling completely demoralized, please be aware that the primary reason for these bad odds is the diets themselves.

The truth is you can lose weight on virtually any diet. Yes, it may be bad for your health and you may be half-starving, but you will drop the pounds if you manage to stick to it. The problem is that almost all diets—unlike the

G.I. Diet—are completely unsustainable. And research tells us that there are three fundamental reasons why:

1. The diets are too complicated, written in incomprehensible jargon, and requiring dieters to count calories and measure and weigh portions.
2. The diets leave people feeling hungry and deprived all the time and unwilling to continue.
3. The diets make people feel unwell because the regimens are having a negative impact on their health. Many, if not most, diets are potentially damaging to one's health.

Clearly, it's pretty impossible to stick to a diet with any of the above characteristics. That's why I deliberately constructed the G.I. Diet to deal with each of those problems head on. First, the program is simplicity itself. You don't have to figure out the number of calories in everything you eat. If you can follow a traffic light, you can follow this diet. Second, if you eat all the recommended meals and snacks, you will not go hungry or feel deprived. This is the core reason why people are able to stick to this diet. Third, this program will not only do no harm to your health, it will actually benefit it. Because the G.I. Diet includes whole grains, fruits and vegetables, low-fat dairy products, protein and beneficial fats, it will actually improve your odds against today's major diseases, such as heart disease and stroke, diabetes, Alzheimer's and many forms of cancer. In summary then, the G.I. Diet addresses all the principal reasons why most diets don't work. And I guarantee that you will feel better on this diet than you ever have before.

This may be hard to believe, but when I reached my target weight after losing twenty-two pounds, I had to make a conscious effort to eat more in order to avoid losing more weight. My wife said I was entering "the gaunt zone"! In Phase II, you must eat more than you did during the weight-loss portion of the diet in order to maintain your new weight. Remember the equation: food energy ingested must equal energy expended to keep weight stable. But I do have a few words of caution. You will require considerably less calories than you did before you started the diet because first, your body has become accustomed to doing with fewer calories and has to a certain extent adapted. Your body is more efficient than it was in the bad old days. Second, your slimmer body needs fewer calories to function. For example, if you lost 10 percent of your body weight, you now require 10 percent fewer calories.

The biggest mistake most people make when coming off a diet is to assume they can go back to eating the way they did before the diet. The reality is that you will probably need only a marginal increase in food energy to balance out the energy in/energy out equation. Only you can determine how big that increase should be. Try serving yourself slightly larger portion sizes or adding foods from the yellow-light category to your meals. Continue to monitor your weight each week, and if you start to gain, cut down a bit on the yellow-light foods; if you continue to lose, eat a bit more; if your weight remains stable, you've reached that magic balance and this is how you will eat for the rest of your life. You'll know what

Dear Rick,

This is a fabulous diet, if you can call it a diet. I find it's simply a different way of eating—a very simple, common-sense way of eating. For years, I've been slowly putting on weight and wondering why, and then this book explained it to me. I'd become a carbohydrate addict and was constantly eating processed foods. I've always tried to eat healthily and was even vegetarian for several years, but I found that I slowly but surely kept putting on weight. Then I happened to pick up *The G.I. Diet* in a bookstore and started flipping through it. Everything in it made so much sense.

So far, I've been on this so-called diet for just over a month, and have lost 15 pounds. I'm 5' 11" and was at 205 pounds—on the verge of being obese. Now I'm down to 190 pounds and I haven't even started to exercise. . . . My eating habits have changed significantly. I think the biggest thing this diet has given me is the ability to tell when I'm full. I used to overeat all the time because I didn't really feel full. Now I pretty much always feel full, even when it's time to eat—and it takes a heck of a lot less for me to feel full.

I'm at the point now where if I try to indulge myself by having a treat, I pretty much always find it a letdown because my tastes have changed. I firmly believe that not all diets work for all people, but this one definitely works for me!

Phil

your body needs and you won't have to weigh yourself so often. You'll experience none of those hypoglycemic lows and will no longer crave junk food. And you'll be able to cheat once in a while without gaining any pounds. You will be in control of your weight.

Here are some suggestions for how you might wish to modify your eating pattern in Phase II.

Breakfast
- Increase cereal serving size, e.g., from ½ to ⅔ cup oatmeal.
- Add a slice of 100% whole grain toast and a pat of margarine.
- Double up on the sliced almonds on cereals.
- Help yourself to an extra slice of back bacon.
- Have a glass of juice now and then.
- Add one of the forbidden fruits—a banana or a mango—to your cereal.

Lunch
I suggest you continue to eat lunch as you did in Phase I. This is the one meal that contained some compromises in the weight-loss portion of the program since it is a meal that most of us buy each day.

Dinner
- Add another boiled new potato (from two or three to three or four).

- Increase the rice or pasta serving from ¾ to 1 cup.
- Have a 6-ounce steak instead of your regular 4-ounce.
- Eat a few more olives and nuts.
- Try a cob of sweet corn with a dab of non-hydrogenated margarine.
- Have a glass of red wine with dinner.

Snacks

- Have some light microwave popcorn (the maximum serving is 2 cups).
- Indulge in a square or two of bittersweet chocolate (see below).
- Eat a banana.
- Enjoy a scoop of low-fat ice cream.

Chocolate

This rich, luscious treat is the first thing all you choco-holics will want to incorporate back into your diet. And you can. Choose chocolate with a high-cocoa content (a minimum of 70 percent), because it delivers more chocoholic satisfaction per gram, and have only a square or two every once in a while. Because chocolate contains large quantities of saturated fat and sugar, it is quite fattening. But you can definitely get away with a couple of squares. Nibbled slowly or dissolved in the mouth, these two squares are all you'll need to enjoy the taste and get the fix you need.

Alcohol

In Phase II, a daily glass of wine, preferably red and with dinner, is not only allowed, it's encouraged! Red wine is particularly rich in flavonoids, and when it is drunk in moderation (a glass a day), it has a demonstrable benefit in reducing the risk of heart attack and stroke.

What about beer? Well, unfortunately for all us beer aficionados, beer has an exceptionally high G.I. rating due to its malt content. Still, I do enjoy an occasional pint. Real discretion is required here. If you do drink alcohol, always have it with a meal. Food slows down the absorption of alcohol, thereby minimizing its impact.

With all these new options in Phase II, the temptation may be to overdo it. Remember to continue to weigh yourself weekly when you first begin in order to find your equilibrium. Once you do, eating the right amount will become second nature. You will find that Phase II is an easy and quite natural way to live, and that many of those high-fat foods you once thought you couldn't live without are no longer desirable.

Part Two

Living
the G.I. Diet

CHAPTER FIVE

Coach's Corner

By this point it's most likely safe to assume that you've committed yourself to the principles of the G.I. Diet and to losing weight permanently. Perhaps you've completed the five essential steps for getting started and have even begun to lose weight. Maybe you've already been on the diet for a few months and are seeing substantial results. Whatever stage you may be at, you are bound to face the inevitable dieting hurdles that test everyone's firmest resolve. Food cravings, holidays and celebrations, vacations and flagging enthusiasm are all challenges to our commitment to healthy eating. In this chapter, I will give you some tips for dealing with these dietary hazards.

Food Cravings

What makes losing weight particularly challenging is that we tend to enjoy and desire fattening foods such as chocolate, cookies, ice cream, peanut butter, chips and so on. The most important thing to remember about cravings is that we're only human and it's natural to succumb to temptation every now and then. Don't feel guilty about it. If you "cheat," you aren't totally blowing your diet. You're simply experiencing a temporary blip in your good eating habits. If you have a small piece of chocolate cake after dinner, or perhaps a beer with the guys while watching the game, make sure you savour the extravagance by eating or drinking *slowly*. Really enjoy it. Then get back on track in the morning with a green-light breakfast and stick to the straight and narrow for the next couple of weeks. You will continue to lose weight, and that's what it's all about.

A friend of mine, who is a cardiologist, allows himself a few "red days" a month. These are days when he knows he has strayed from the guidelines of the G.I. Diet. To prevent red days from becoming a habit, he monitors them by marking them on his calendar. The G.I. Diet itself will help prevent lapses in two key ways. First, you will find that after you've been on the program for a few weeks, you will have developed a built-in warning system: you won't feel good physically when you eat a red-light food because your blood sugar will spike and crash. You'll feel bloated, uncomfortable and lethargic, and you may even get a headache—a strong deterrent against straying into red-light territory. Second, because you are eating three meals and three snacks daily, you won't feel hungry between meals. If you skip any, you will probably start longing for forbidden foods—so make sure you eat all the recommended meals and snacks every day.

Despite the diet's built-in security system, there will be times when a craving gets the better of you. What should you do? Well, you could try substituting a green-light food for the red-light food you're thinking about. If you want something sweet, try having fruit; applesauce; low-fat,

Dear Rick,

Thank you so much for giving me my life back! When I heard about your book I thought I would give it a go but that it would probably end up on the shelf with all the other diet books I've got. How wrong I was. I was 240 pounds eight weeks ago, and I'm now down to 210 pounds. Amazingly I have dropped two dress sizes. The weird thing is, apart from relinquishing the obligatory spud at every meal, I still feel like I've yet to start the diet!

I feel absolutely wonderful—I have energy to keep going all day without having to nap—and my husband can't keep his hands off me! My doctor is stunned by my progress and is going to start recommending this diet to his other highly obese patients.

After spending most of my life binging, comfort-eating and basically grossly abusing my body, at the age of 32 I think I might possibly find a slim person! I know I have about 56 pounds still to go to be an "acceptable" weight in the stereo-typical way, but this time it doesn't frighten me. Thank you again for helping me to reclaim by life (and my body)!

Maeve

sugar-free yogurt; low-fat ice cream with no added sugar; any of Emily's dessert recipes; a food bar or a caffeine-free diet soft drink. If what you want is something salty and crunchy, try having a dill pickle or Emily's Dried Chickpeas (page 233). You could also make some Sage and Tomato White Bean Dip (page 234) and have it with celery sticks.

Your craving for chocolate in Phase I may be alleviated with a chocolate flavoured food bar, with light instant chocolate or with Emily's Baked Chocolate Mousse (page 251) or Pecan Brownies (page 254). As you can see, there are many green-light versions of the foods we normally reach for when a craving strikes.

Sometimes, however, there isn't a likely substitute for the foods we miss. I have received many e-mails from readers who love peanut butter and say they cannot live without it. The thing to do here is to select the most nutritional product available—the natural kind that is made from peanuts only and has no additives such as sugar—and eat only a tablespoon of it once in a while. It's better to consume the good fats that are in peanuts than the red-light fillers that are found in other varieties of peanut butter. Don't be fooled into thinking the "lite" versions are better for you. The amount of peanuts in these products has been reduced and sugar and starch fillers have been added. Remember that the more red-light foods you consume, the more you will slow your progress in achieving your target BMI.

Holidays and Celebrations

We all know how much determination and gumption it takes to commit ourselves to a new weight-loss plan and how much drive it takes to clear one's cupboards, go shopping and embark on an unfamiliar way of eating. That's why once we have managed to do all this, the last thing we want is for a holiday to come along and throw a wrench into our progress. Christmas, Thanksgiving, Easter, Passover and so on all have one thing in common: an abundance of food. Holidays are generally centred around traditional feasts and dishes. But even so, you don't have to throw the G.I. guidelines out the window. You can stay in the green and still have a fun and festive holiday.

If you host the event yourself, you will be able to decide what type of food is served. Think of what you would normally eat during the holiday and look for green-light alternatives. For example, if you usually have a roast turkey with bread-based stuffing for Thanksgiving, have a roast turkey with wild or basmati rice stuffing instead. If you always make cranberry sauce with sugar, prepare it with a sugar substitute. My wife, Ruth, and I always add slivered almonds and chunks of orange to our cranberry sauce—delicious! There is no shortage of green-light vegetables to serve as side dishes, and dessert can be elegant poached pears or a pavlova with berries. You can put on a completely green-light feast without your guests even realizing.

If you celebrate the holiday at someone else's home, you will obviously have less control over the menu. You could help out the busy host by offering to bring a vegetable side dish or the dessert—a green-light one, of course. Once seated at the holiday table, survey the dishes and try to compose your plate as you would at home: vegetables on half the plate, rice or pasta on one quarter and a source of protein on the other. Pass on the rolls and mashed potatoes—have extra vegetables instead. If you wish, you can allow yourself a concession by having a small serving of dessert. If you aren't particularly big on sweets, you might prefer to have a glass of wine instead. Try not to indulge in both.

Cocktail parties can also be fun, green-light occasions. Instead of alcohol, you can have a glass of mineral water with a twist of lemon or a diet caffeine-free soft drink. If you really would like an alcoholic beverage, have only one and try to choose the least red-light option. Red wine is your best bet, or a white wine spritzer made half with wine and half with sparkling water. Be sure to consume any alcohol with food to slow down the rate at which you metabolize it. Beer has a very high G.I. rating, so that's a real concession. Have it if you really want it, but make sure it's only one. Other drinks are also high G.I. and high calorie.

If you host the cocktail party yourself, you can make all the appetizers green-light. Have a cooked, sliced turkey as a centrepiece and offer lean sliced deli ham with a selection of mustards. Serve a variety of raw vegetables with a choice of low-fat dips and salsa. Hummus with wedges of whole wheat pita, smoked salmon or caviar on cucumber slices, crab salad on snow peas, chicken or beef skewers, meatballs made with extra-lean ground beef, and sashimi with soy sauce all make wonderful appetizers that everyone will enjoy. You can also provide bowls of nuts and olives, but remember to have only a few of each and don't linger nearby—it's too tempting to keep munching as you chat with your guests. Be sure to also serve a platter piled decoratively with a wide variety of green-light fruits.

If you are attending someone else's cocktail party, have a green-light meal before you go so you won't be tempted to eat too much. Then choose the low-G.I. appetizers and enjoy your time with friends and family.

Vacations and Dining Out

Going away on vacation usually means having to eat all your meals at restaurants—unless you spend a week at a cottage or a beach house where you can do the cooking yourself. It's not terribly difficult, though, to put the G.I. guidelines into practice when dining out. First of all, you must ask the server not to leave the habitual basket of bread or rolls on your table. If it's not there, you won't be tempted.

Order a green salad to start and choose a low-fat dressing to be served on the side so that you can control the amount you use. Salads have a very low-G.I. rating (if made with low-G.I. ingredients) and will help to fill you up before the main course arrives, so you won't be tempted to overeat. Then order an entree that includes a low-fat source of protein. Since boiled new potatoes are rarely available and you may not be sure what sort of rice is being used, ask for double the amount of vegetables instead. I've made this request in hundreds of restaurants and have never been refused. On page 269, I have included a detachable summary of dining out tips that you can keep in your wallet or purse.

When the server brings you the healthy, green-light meal you ordered, be sure to eat it slowly. There is a distinct connection between the speed at which we eat our food and feeling full or satiated. The stomach can take twenty to thirty minutes to let the brain know when it feels full. So you may be shovelling in more food than you require before your brain says stop. The other day, a friend of mine, who is a physician, noted that one of the common traits among his overweight physician colleagues was that they tended to bolt down their food. He thought that the habit probably stemmed from the days when they were busy residents and had to eat as quickly as they could in the hectic hospital environment. The famous Dr. Samuel Johnson in the eighteenth century advised chewing food thirty-two times before swallowing it! That's probably going overboard, but at least put your fork down between mouthfuls. If you savour your food by eating more slowly, you will leave the table feeling far more satisfied—you'll be amazed at the difference it makes.

Just because you are on vacation doesn't mean you shouldn't continue to eat three meals and three snacks daily. In your suitcase, pack some green-light snacks to take with you, such as food bars, nuts and any other non-perishables. Once there, you can buy non-fat, sugar-free yogurt, fruit, low-fat cottage cheese and applesauce to snack on. Avoid the Continental breakfasts offered in some hotels. They are generally made up of red-light foods and offer little in the way of nutrition. One option for breakfast is to buy your own fruit, green-light cereals and milk at a supermarket and have breakfast in your hotel room.

If you are driving to your destination or are going on a road trip, your only option along the highway may be fast food. If you can, pack some green-light meals and snacks to take with you, so you won't have to stop to eat. Otherwise, I have provided some tips for eating at fast food outlets on pages 38 to 39.

Staying Motivated

Losing weight takes time and patience. If it took you five years to gain twenty pounds, how can you expect to lose them in the space of a month? Most people tend to lose the first few pounds very quickly. But as your body adjusts to the new way of eating, you may have a week where you won't lose, while other weeks you may lose two or three pounds. Remember that it's the average that counts, and you should target an average of *one pound per week*. How do you stay motivated for the time it takes to reach your BMI target? In my first book, *The G.I. Diet*, I listed a number of tips that are worth repeating here.

1. Maintain your weekly progress log. Success is a powerful motivator.
2. Set up a reward system. Buy yourself a small gift when you achieve a predetermined weight goal—perhaps a gift for every three pounds lost.
3. Identify family members or friends who will be your cheerleaders. Make them active participants in your plan. Even better, find a friend who will join the plan for mutual support.
4. Avoid acquaintances and haunts that may encourage your old behaviours. You know who I mean!
5. Try adding what my wife, Ruth, calls a special "spa" day to your week—a day when you are especially good with your program. This will give you some extra credit in your weight-loss account to draw on when the inevitable relapse occurs.
6. Check out **www.gidiet.com** to read about other dieters' experiences, to share your own and to keep updated on new developments.

Your Health

If your enthusiasm starts to flag, try to remember what you were thinking and feeling the day you decided to start the G.I. Diet. You were probably feeling fed up and wishing you were slim. You were probably concerned about your health, too. And you had good reason to be. The fatter you are, the more likely it is that you will suffer a heart attack or stroke, develop diabetes and raise your risk for many cancers.

The two key factors linking heart disease and stroke to diet are cholesterol and hypertension (high blood pressure). High cholesterol is the key ingredient in the plaque that can build up in your arteries, eventually cutting off the supply of blood to your heart (causing heart attack) or your brain (leading to stroke). Hypertension puts more stress on the arterial system, causing it to age and deteriorate more rapidly, ultimately leading to arterial damage, blood clots, and heart attack or stroke. Excess weight has a major bearing on high blood pressure. A Canadian study in 1997 found that obese adults, aged eighteen to fifty-five, had a five- to thirteen-times greater risk of hypertension.

Diabetes is the kissing cousin of heart disease in that more people die from heart complications arising from diabetes than from diabetes alone. And diabetes rates are skyrocketing: they are expected to double in the next ten years. The principal causes of the most common form of diabetes, Type 2, are obesity and lack of exercise, and the current epidemic is strongly correlated to the obesity trend.

Being overweight has also been linked to cancer. A recent global report by the American Institute for Cancer Research concluded that 30 to 40 percent of cancers are directly linked to dietary choices. Its key recommendation is that individuals should choose a predominantly plant-based diet that includes a variety of vegetables, fruits and whole grains—basically what the G.I. Diet recommends. So please do stick with it. Your weight has tremendous bearing on your health. What's worth more to you, a hamburger and fries or a long, healthy life to be shared with loved ones? I think the choice is obvious.

Dear Rick,

I am writing this testimonial to your diet on behalf of my mother who is 79 years young and very grateful for your book. She was diagnosed with diabetes last spring. . . and was a candidate for a heart attack. She was very worried. Her doctor gave her six months to do something about it through diet and exercise before putting her on insulin. He prescribed your book and wished her luck.

She was so afraid of having to take insulin every day that she was really motivated to follow your recommendations. She did so faithfully and has lost 23 pounds! More importantly, her blood sugar has gone down to 4. . . . She is completely convinced of the value of your program and tells everyone about it. . . . From my perspective, as a daughter who cherishes her mom, I can't tell you how happy it makes me when my mother shows me yet another garment that needs to be made smaller because of her success. Her pride and sense of accomplishment only enhance an already special lady, and I thank you for it.

Monique

CHAPTER SIX

The G.I. Family

As I mentioned in the previous chapter, one way of staying motivated on the G.I. Diet is to get a family member on board. If both of you are trying to lose weight together, you can support each other and have fun while doing so. More often than not, the letters I receive tell me about the results both husband and wife are seeing now that they're on the program together. But not everyone has someone in his or her family who wants or needs to lose weight. Does that mean they have to prepare separate meals for themselves? The answer is absolutely not.

The G.I. Diet is suitable for the whole family because it's really not a diet at all—it's simply a very healthy way of eating, based on real, everyday foods. Phase II is the way we should eat throughout our entire lives. A friend of mine who went on the G.I. Diet began serving herself and her husband green-light meals for dinner every night without telling him they were based on the G.I. guidelines. He never even realized he was eating according to the recommendations of a diet plan!

Phase II is also an ideal way for children to eat—and not just those who need to lose weight. We all know that the number of overweight and obese Canadians has risen dramatically in the last several years due to poor eating habits and lack of physical activity. Unfortunately, being overweight has become all too common among children. More than one-third of Canadian kids are overweight and about half of those are obese. That's why it's so important to start introducing good eating habits to your children early on—it will serve them well in the future. Don't you wish you had never been introduced to junk food? If you had never had it, you wouldn't miss it now. If children don't get used to sugary soft drinks and candy, they won't develop cravings for these things later on.

We have found in our home that kids adapt easily to the G.I. way of eating. They like green-light foods and don't feel deprived. Of course, this doesn't mean that your children shouldn't be allowed to enjoy their Halloween treats or birthday cake and ice cream. It's just that these things should be saved for special occasions. On the average day, children should eat a nutritious breakfast (not sugary cereals or Pop Tarts!), lunch and dinner and snacks based on the G.I. guidelines. Fresh fruit, vegetables, fish, chicken, yogurt, whole wheat bread, porridge, and apple bran muffins are all kid-friendly food. Just remember that growing children need sufficient fat in their diet—the good kind of fat found in fish, nuts and vegetable oils.

From the beginning, we made a point of serving our children healthy meals and snacks. We didn't keep soft drinks and other junk food in the house, but we didn't try to police our children either. Halloween always meant a period of "sugar shock," and birthday cakes were always decorated with Smarties. But the rest of the party food we served was nutritious—sandwiches made with whole wheat bread, vegetables with dips, and fruit—and loot bags contained little candy if any. Our son David loved having porridge and yogurt for breakfast, although the consistency of it was always a matter of much negotiation: not too lumpy, not too smooth. We always tried to sit down for dinner as a family and catch up on what was happening with everyone. We never used dessert to bribe them to eat, and we usually served fruit for that course.

Our boys participated in making nutritious snacks. We have photos of the early muffin-makers replete with long aprons and large wooden spoons. They also enjoyed having raw vegetables for snacks if they were accompanied by interesting, low-fat dips. Now as adults, our sons continue to eat healthy diets and do not suffer from cravings for sweets or fast food. They love seafood, eat a wide variety of vegetables and like to introduce their parents to new green-light foods. We first tried edamame pods at my eldest son's home.

So if you haven't yet done so, try serving all your family members green- and yellow-light meals. Don't tell them that they are following the G.I. Diet, just say that you'd like everyone to try eating a healthier way. The early experiences children have with food have tremendous impact on the way they will eat as adults—a trend that my wife, Ruth, happens to know a great deal about. She is a professor at the University of Toronto and specializes in childhood trauma and its effects on behaviour later in life. In the next chapter, she will talk about the role food plays in our upbringing and how we learn to comfort ourselves with it.

Dear Rick,

As a teenager I know that dieting is a big thing for a lot of us. So many of my friends are always trying different diets to lose weight and usually end up going hungry. Because I've witnessed this happen so many times, the idea of dieting completely turned me off—until I found your diet. Considering this was the first diet I'd really ever done, I'm surprised that it actually worked. I've been so amazed with the results, I don't want to give away my secret to my friends! I've managed to lose 24 pounds in a healthy, natural way—even my doctor is pleased with what I have done.

I just wanted to commend you on this wonderful diet. Trust me, I'm never hungry.

Erika

CHAPTER SEVEN

Food as Comfort

As soon as we are born, food and comfort become permanently intertwined. From the moment we are held secure by our mothers and fed snug in their arms, food will always be connected with being held, being safe and being comforted. And these connections stay with us for the rest of our lives.

As we grow, food continues to play a vital role in our relationship with our parents, especially our mothers, since they traditionally have been the preparers of food. Their success or failure as mothers is often judged by the plumpness of their children. Thin babies are considered "malnourished" and, even worse, "neglected" and "uncared for" by a not-good-enough mother. A plump baby with lots of cheek to pinch is perceived as a sign of successful mothering.

As we grew, our milestones were marked by celebrations and parties all based around food. Even when we were ill, Mom could be trusted to make a special effort to feed us foods that would encourage our appetites. When we ourselves became parents, we used food, candy or visits to fastfood restaurants to bribe our children to be good on outings and as rewards for toilet training. Our parents became eager-to-please grandparents who "spoiled" their grandchildren with an apparent bottomless pit of food goodies.

Food permeates all aspects of our social life. It plays a role far beyond nourishing us and ensuring our continued survival. Food is a way for us to show trust, friendship and love. We celebrate holidays, such as Thanksgiving, Christmas, Passover and Easter, with food. From christenings and circumcisions to funerals and wakes, food is the one constant companion throughout our lives. In some cultures, the "breaking of bread" together symbolizes trust, and to refuse food when offered would be perceived as an insult. As we venture forth into the world, food continues to take a central place in our social activities, such as dating and "doing lunch" for business or pleasure. And what would a football game be without beer and pizza?

Our relationship with food, however, isn't always wonderful. Food can also be used as a weapon. Children use it as a way of rebelling against their family. Most of you can probably remember the endless battle of wills to get children to eat, often ending with food being choked down or spit up. Our youngest son went through an "only bananas and yogurt" phase that seemed to go on for an age but likely lasted only a week—we all survived without serious consequence. And the games we played to persuade them to eat! I can remember cutting toast into strips, dipping them into the required food at hand and flying them with aircraft sounds into our son's waiting airplane hangar (mouth). The associations we make between food and the people we love are a critical part of our developmental history.

Food can also be used to induce guilt. While the popular media make jokes about the Jewish/Greek/Italian mother who forcefeeds her children in a display of love, the message "if you love me, you will eat my food" can be a burden. Not being able to leave the table until the overflowing food on the plate is eaten or being unable to refuse a second helping without "hurting" the feelings of Mother can establish habits of overeating as well as conflicting feelings around food for a lifetime. Rick, for example, was taught to always eat everything on his plate and to this day finds it hard not to clean it up along with everything on the table. As a result, I have learned not to put out an excess of food—just the right amount.

Like Rick, we bring to our eating habits our unique history of early experiences and associations with food. When I'm ill, I like chicken soup with rice or tomato soup with macaroni because that's what my much-loved grandmother would feed me as a child. The soup thus comforts my stomach and my psyche, unconsciously reviving the good feelings I felt in the cared-for presence of my grandmother. This kind of connection between food and psychological nurturing is common and not something we do consciously. I don't think about my grandmother every time I eat chicken soup, but I sure feel better.

We also bring other kinds of eating habits with us. As children, many of us would come home from school and head straight to the kitchen for a snack. Now as adults, we may still head for the kitchen as soon as we come home— not just to make dinner but to have a snack. Given the hectic pace of our lives—working full time as well as somehow fitting in ferrying our children to and from child care, shopping, going to dentist appointments and so on—the ritual of walking in the door and reaching for food may be the only time during the entire day when we do something just for ourselves! Due to my British heritage, I like to come home and have a cup of tea with my afternoon green-light snack before starting the "evening shift." It's important to me that I always sit down and have this snack even if it's only for five minutes (it's five minutes for *me*).

Now, while we all use food as comfort or a reward to a greater or lesser extent, for some of us it can become a too-important comforter in our lives. This can put us at serious risk for overeating, weight gain and obesity. Of course there are other ways to soothe ourselves by putting things in our mouth—smoking, drinking and doing drugs being other key self-soothing behaviours. Many of these behaviours can become habits. Just as we can get into the habit of smoking, we can get into the habit of sitting down to watch television with food in hand—and as we all know, breaking a habit is very hard to do.

If you are in the habit of frequent snack eating, giving up those comfort foods is going to be a challenge, particularly since comfort foods are often junk foods, such as chips, cookies and candies, which have a high G.I. rating and therefore provide a quick sugar rush that feels good briefly. These foods do nothing to really fill you up either psychologically or physiologically and generally only leave you craving more. And so the vicious cycle continues, leaving you feeling even unhappier because of the weight gain that results.

This doesn't mean you can't snack—far from it. The G.I. Diet recommends having three snacks a day in addition to your regular three meals. It's just that your snacks are going to be different. Choose fruit, a whole range of low-fat dairy products, and homemade muesli and muffins, just to name a few options. Until you get into the habit of eating this way, these snacks may not provide the sugar rush "comfort" and mouth-feel you rely on to feel good. So it may be helpful to start thinking about alternative ways to comfort yourself when alone in the evening after a hard day at work.

Take some time to think about how and when you eat. Do you eat on the run, standing up, taking little or no real pleasure in your eating? Are meals enjoyable social times or times of high stress and tension? Do you walk in the door after work and start eating continuously until bedtime, and are you aware you are doing this? When you really think about it, are you eating for reasons other than to alleviate hunger? Do you eat to relieve boredom, stress, anxiety or loneliness?

If this sounds like you, then you need to stop and think: are there things you can change so that mealtimes are pleasurable and tension free? Take some time to plan your meals (consider weekly meal plans) and make time for shopping and preparation. Next try to ensure that you always sit down at a table at a fairly regular time to eat your meals. Don't eat standing up or while doing other chores or tasks. Relax and enjoy your food, eating slowly. Once you have thought about ways to make meals comforting and enjoyable, you can start thinking about how you can substitute pleasurable activities for some of your snacking habits. To do this, I'd like you to draw up a list of all the

activities you enjoy doing, including hobbies and pleasurable distractions. I've included an example of a list
below, but yours will be unique to you.

Activities
Having a bath surrounded by candles
Listening to music
Going to a baseball game
Doing yoga
Going to see a movie
Hiking in the outdoors
Woodworking
Calling a friend
Fishing
Looking at old photographs
Reading a novel
Making a scrapbook
Writing a diary

Doing some of the items on your list may feel self-indulgent
and a waste of time—something we've been taught is a bad
thing. It's okay, a good idea even, to do pleasurable, nice
things for yourself.

So the next time you feel like reaching for a red-light
snack, perhaps a bowl of popcorn while watching television, do one of the activities on your list instead. Have a
warm bubble bath or call a friend to chat. I know this shift
sounds hard, but take it slowly and remember that the first
step to any kind of change is recognizing that something
needs to change. By reading this book, you've already

started that process. If you have a partner, get him or her on side—the support of friends and family is essential if this is going to really work. Make sure they understand what you are trying to do and get them to help you by including them in your activities.

Food will always play an important part in our lives as a source of nutrition, in socialization and for comfort. Eating can be pleasurable and satisfying. By slowly making healthy changes to the way you eat, you will find that food has a more balanced place in your life.

> Dear Rick,
>
> I wanted to write and thank you for your book. I have been overweight all my life. . . . I had peaked at 302 pounds and had come to the conclusion that I was a food addict and that trying to lose weight was hopeless, having tried every other plan out there—or so I thought!
>
> Thank God a very dear friend of mine found your book. Seven weeks later I weigh 273 pounds and have never felt so good. Your plan has turned off my inner demon's voice! I no longer crave sweet things . . . I haven't had ANY chocolate in seven weeks (the longest I have been without it since birth, I swear!) and I am finding the plan easy to stick to and easy to manage. Now thanks to you I KNOW I am going to get down to a healthy body weight for the first time in my life. I am 37 years old and I feel like my life is just starting. Thank you, thank you, thank you!!
>
> Sarah

CHAPTER EIGHT

Frequently Asked Questions

Q. Can I really eat as much of the green-light foods as I want?

A. Yes you can, except where I recommend a specific serving or portion size. Serving sizes are important for green-light foods that have a higher G.I. rating or calorie content than others, such as pasta, rice, bread, nuts and meat. Let common sense be your guide and keep everything in moderation. I wouldn't recommend eating twenty oranges a day, for example, or ten green-light muffins. That's going a bit overboard.

Q. Is there any flexibility in this diet?

A. Yes, but only you can determine which rules you can break and still lose weight. Many readers tell me they can't live without certain red-light foods such as regular coffee or peanut butter. If there's a product that is that important to you, go ahead and have it, but strictly limit the quantity you consume. Have only one cup of coffee or one tablespoon of peanut butter a day. One reader told me she was on the "Vegas" version of the G.I. Diet, meaning she had a glass of red wine every day on Phase I. She still lost thirty pounds and is wearing the same dress size she wore back in university. Although you would lose weight faster if you followed all the guidelines of the G.I. Diet, it really is okay to live only 90 percent on the program.

Q. I thought aspartame and some other sugar substitutes were bad for your health, so why are you recommending them?

A. A great deal of misinformation has been spread about sugar substitutes—driven mainly by the sugar lobby in the United States. All the major government and health agencies worldwide have approved the use of sweeteners and sugar substitutes and not a single peer-reviewed (scholarly) study has identified any health risks. For those who are still concerned about the safety of artificial sweeteners, there is a comprehensive rundown on sugar substitutes in the U.S. Food and Drug Administration Consumer Magazine (see www.fda.gov).

If you're sensitive to aspartame, check out the alternatives such as sucralose (Splenda) or saccharine (Sweet 'n Low).

Q. Is the herbal sweetener stevia a green-light product?

A. Stevia is a South American herb that can be found in health stores. Although its popularity is growing, no long-term studies on its safety have been carried out—so I can't wholeheartedly recommend it. But it appears to be an acceptable alternative if used in moderation.

Q. I understand that peanut butter has a low G.I. If so, why is it red-light? Are the "lite" versions more acceptable?

A. It's true that peanut butter has a low G.I. rating, but it is extremely high in fat and is calorie dense. Unfortunately, the "lite" varieties are even worse because the amount of peanuts has been reduced and sugar and starch fillers have been added to make up the shortfall. If you are going to "cheat" with an occasional tablespoon of peanut butter, make sure it's the natural kind that contains 100 percent peanuts and no added sugar.

Q. Beans are listed as green-light, yet commercially canned black bean soup is red-light. Why?

A. Beans are a classic green-light food, low in fat and high in protein and fibre. Commercially canned bean soups, however, are highly processed and therefore high-G.I. They are cooked at extremely high temperatures to prevent spoilage. This process breaks down both the outer protective skin of the beans and the starch granules inside—something that would normally be done by your digestive system. Because of this, canned black bean, split pea and green pea soups are all high-G.I. Try Emily's homemade bean soups instead, which are green-light and easy to make.

Q. Dried apricots and cranberries are listed as yellow-light yet they are used in some green-light recipes. Don't they raise the G.I. level of the recipes?

A. Dried fruits actually have a low-G.I. They are for the most part, however, high in calories, which is why most are listed in the red-light column. Dried apricots and cranberries have a lower calorie content, and the amount used in the recipes is so modest, they only marginally raise the calorie content, not enough to worry about.

Q. I know you should avoid drinking alcohol in Phase I, but can you use wine in recipes?

A. Absolutely! You can cook with wine even in Phase I. Adding a cup to a sauce that is going to serve four people means that each person will only be getting a quarter cup—much less than a glass of wine. Also, most of the alcohol tends to evaporate in the cooking process.

Q. Are low-calorie foods such as rice cakes or sugar-free Jell-O green-light foods?

A. I'm afraid not. Although they don't have a lot of calories, they are digested quickly, leaving you looking for more food to keep your digestive system busy. Try to stick to green-light snacks, which are far more nutritious and satisfying.

Q. I read that many high-fat foods such as premium ice cream are in fact low-G.I. Is this true?

A. Yes it is. Fat acts as a brake on the digestive process, which means that fatty foods take longer to digest. But they are still red-light for two reasons. First, they are high in calories. Fat contains more than twice the calories per gram than protein or carbohydrates. Second, most high-fat foods contain saturated fats, which are bad for your health. Though the G.I. content of foods is a very important factor in determining whether a food is green-light or not, we must also take into account its calorie density and its impact on our health. Saturated fat is definitely a bad fat.

Dear Rick,

Thank you for your continued work with the G.I. program. I started in May, went great guns for a while and hit a plateau. Your book has changed the way I think about food and my plateau has started to crumble again and the pounds are coming off—slowly, just the way they should. I have lost 13 pounds and I look and feel so much better. I still have a long way to go. My goal is another 20 pounds over the next two years.

My heart, my body and my soul thank you for your motivation and support.

Take care,

Glennda

Q. I've been on the G.I. Diet for several weeks and have been very pleased with my progress until the last couple of weeks or so. I seem to have hit a plateau. What should I do?

A. Most people experience rapid weight loss during the first few weeks of the diet. That sets up the expectation that weight loss will continue at the same rate, but this is generally not the case. You should expect to lose an average of one pound per week. Don't be overly concerned if you hit a plateau. If you are following the G.I. Diet guidelines and are still above your recommended BMI, you will definitely reach your goal. If your plateau seems to be lasting a bit too long, think about what you have been eating lately and whether you may be straying a bit too far from the green-light column of the food guide. I received an e-mail from a reader who said he had reached a plateau and that his only indiscretion was a couple of peanut butter snacks a day. Well, the problem was that this "indiscretion" was delivering about 3,500 calories, or a pound of fat, to his waistline every week. No wonder he had hit a plateau!

PART THREE

Cooking the
G.I. Way

CHAPTER NINE

Introduction to G.I. Cooking

When Rick first approached me to put together a collection of recipes for his best-selling diet, I was delighted. I've always been interested in healthy cooking (I have a degree in nutrition) and have developed countless low-fat recipes for Canadian Living over the years. Rick told me that not only would the recipes for this book have to be low in saturated fat, but they'd also have to be high fibre, low in sugar, have a low G.I. rating—and oh, taste great, too. I told him to sign me up right away! I love to create new recipes because it allows me to express my passion for cooking while "playing" in the kitchen. And I would be helping out not only all you G.I. dieters, but also some of my own family members who have been diagnosed with diabetes, high cholesterol, high blood pressure and heart disease.

When you first begin the G.I. Diet, you may feel as though there are a lot of limitations on what you can eat. But focus on what's listed in the green-light column of the food guide, and you will see that there really is a wide-ranging variety of appealing foods. You can eat very well on the G.I. Diet and never have to sacrifice flavour. Not only are green-light foods good for you, but I also happen to think that they are some of the best tasting. Extra-virgin olive oil, for example, is a monounsaturated, or "best," fat and adds a wonderful flavour to many dishes.

Good taste is always my primary consideration when developing new recipes. I start with my own personal experiences with food—what I enjoy cooking and what my family and friends take pleasure in eating. I like to use plenty of fresh herbs, delicious spices and ethnic flavours to come up with interesting and fun meals. In this collection, you will find some old family favourites, such as Veal Parmesan and Beef Fajitas, that I have modified to make green-light. By using less oil, avoiding white flour and sugar and using strong cheeses for flavour enhancement only, you too can turn your own much-loved recipes into green-light dishes. Ruth and Rick have shared a few of their standbys, and thanks to your e-mails, there are some readers' recipes here, too.

Cooking the G.I. way generally means cooking from scratch and avoiding heavily processed foods. But that doesn't mean you have to spend a lot of time in the kitchen. Most of the recipes in this book can be made in less than thirty minutes. I've included some breakfast recipes, such as Yogurt Smoothies and Muesli, for those mornings when you are on the run, as well as some recipes that are more suited for relaxing weekends, like Light 'n' Fluffy Pancakes and Back Bacon Omelette. Any of the salad and soup recipes will form the basis of a satisfying lunch, and there are plenty of meatless, fish and seafood, poultry and meat dishes to choose from for dinner. And because this isn't a deprivation diet, I've also included some recipes for desserts and snacks that I'm sure you will enjoy. I've tried almost all of them out on my family, friends and cooking classes, and everyone has been amazed to discover that they are low fat and low G.I.—they taste that good. I hope that many of these green- and yellow-light dishes will become favourites among your own family and friends. In the following sections, I have included some tips on ingredients, equipment, measuring and side dishes, and have given you a week-long menu plan to help you get started.

Dear Rick,

I just wanted you to know that I saw your interview with Vicki Gabereau earlier today. My daughter and I started the G.I. Diet a couple months ago, and I have lost 16 pounds and my daughter has lost almost the same . . . We love the food! Old habits are certainly hard to change, but having food prepared ahead of time sure makes a difference when one is short on time. If I make batches of soup, chili and granola bars, I can be very good. However, if I haven't made some things ahead of time, it is soooo easy to fall back on old familiar (but harmful) eating patterns!

The big discovery for me was to find out how awful I feel when I go off your plan and start grabbing sweets or some such thing for a day! Y-U-C-K. I can't believe that I used to feel like that all the time before your book! I never would have thought that yogurt would become such a good friend.

Thanks again,

Bernice

Ingredients

You will notice that not all of the ingredients that I have used in the recipes are strictly green-light. I've added wine for depth of flavour, as well as small amounts of sauces that contain sugar, and dried fruit. This doesn't mean that the recipe is yellow- or red-light. The quantities are so minor that they will have little to no effect on your blood sugar level. Don't feel you have to omit them to stay in the green.

To replace sugar in recipes, I've had great success with Splenda and Sugar Twin and have found the flavour quite good. Look for the granular type that comes in boxes because it is the easiest to use—you can measure out the amount just like sugar.

Equipment

Non-stick skillets

When cooking low-fat dishes, it's useful to have a few non-stick skillets on hand in various sizes. You only need a minimal amount of oil when using them and food slides right off the pan. Remember that the recommended cooking heat for non-stick surfaces is no higher than medium-high and that you should use non-abrasive utensils and brushes only. Wash your skillet with hot soapy water and a nylon brush—do not put it in the dishwasher, which will damage the non-stick coating. If you need to stick your skillet in the oven and it has a plastic or wood handle, be sure to wrap the handle well with aluminum foil first. And if there is wear and tear on your pans, consider buying new ones for better performance.

Grill pan/Indoor grill

The tips I gave above for caring for your non-stick pans also apply to grill pans and indoor grills. When using them, you only need a light brush or spray of oil. A grill pan keeps the food you are cooking out of the fat and gives that grilled look when you don't have an outdoor barbecue.

Pots and pans

Ever wondered what the difference is between a pot and a pan? Well, a pot usually has two handles and a pan has only one. They can pretty much be used interchangeably. A Dutch oven is just a large pan or pot that has a lid—most people have one without even realizing it!

Measuring

To ensure success with these recipes, be sure to use measuring cups and spoons. Use wet measuring cups, which are usually glass or plastic and have a pouring spout, to measure milk, juice, stock and water. Look at the wet ingredients at eye level on a flat surface for correct measurements. Use dry measuring cups, which are plastic or metal and nest inside each other, to measure flour, sugar, pasta and anything with a thick consistency like sour cream and margarine. Dry ingredients are measured by spooning into the measuring cup and levelling it off with the back of a knife without tapping or adding more. Measuring spoons are usually metal or plastic and can be used for both wet and dry ingredients. You should also level off measuring spoons with a flat surface.

A kitchen scale can be very useful when weighing pasta, meat, vegetables and fruit. Look for one with a bowl or container on top for ease of measuring. If you don't have a scale and you'd like to measure out 6 ounces of long pasta—which is what I've used in the recipes in this book—simply grab a handful of spaghetti or linguine tightly and squeeze into a bundle. It should have the same circumference as a loonie or measure 1 inch across.

Side Dishes

Almost all of the dinner recipes I have included in this book should be accompanied by side dishes. A quarter of your plate should be filled with a starchy carbohydrate such as pasta, rice or boiled new potatoes. Since overcooking tends to raise the G.I. level of food, boil pasta until it is just "al dente," or still firm when bitten, and take rice off the heat before it starts to clump together. Small new potatoes will only take about ten minutes to boil or steam.

Half your plate should be filled with green-light vegetables and salad. Again, do not overcook the veggies; they should be tender-crisp. Most people I know are not avid fans of mushy, flavourless vegetables anyway. Here are some hints for preparing your side vegetables.

Vegetable Steaming Chart

Vegetable	Preparation
Asparagus	trim ends
Broccoli	cut into florets
Brussels sprouts	trim and halve
Carrots	cut into ½-inch chunks
Cauliflower	cut into florets
Frozen green peas	do not thaw
Frozen mixed vegetables in bags	do not thaw
Green beans	trim tips
New potatoes	scrub and prick with fork
Snow peas/sugar snap peas	trim tips
Yellow beans	trim tips
Zucchini	cut into chunks

You can cook these vegetables in any of the following ways.

To boil vegetable: In a saucepan of boiling water, cook vegetable for about 7 minutes or until it is tender-crisp.

To steam vegetable: In a saucepan, boil 1 inch of water. Place steamer basket filled with vegetable in saucepan. Cover with lid and steam for 5 to 7 minutes or until vegetable is tender-crisp.

To microwave vegetable: Place vegetable in large plate or bowl. Add ¼ cup of water. Cover with plastic wrap and microwave on High for about 5 minutes or until vegetable is tender-crisp. To dress up and add some zing to vegetables, drizzle with lemon juice and add salt and pepper.

Salads

The following recipe makes a good basic salad and vinaigrette that you can endlessly vary by using different vegetables, vinegars and herbs.

Basic Salad

1½ cups	lettuce (such as romaine, mesclun, leaf, Boston, arugula, watercress, iceberg)
1	small carrot, shredded
Half	bell pepper (red, yellow or green)
1	plum tomato, cut in wedges
½ cup	sliced cucumber
¼ cup	sliced red onion (optional)

In bowl, toss together lettuce, carrot, bell pepper, tomato, cucumber and onion. Makes 1 serving.

Basic Vinaigrette

1 tbsp	vinegar (such as white or red wine, balsamic, rice or cider) or lemon juice
1 tsp	extra virgin olive or canola oil
½ tsp	Dijon mustard
Pinch	each salt and pepper
Pinch	dried or fresh herb of choice (such as thyme, oregano, basil, Italian seasoning, marjoram, mint)

In small bowl, whisk together vinegar, oil, mustard, salt, pepper and herb. Pour dressing over greens and toss. Makes enough for 1 serving.

A Sample One-Week Green-Light Menu Plan

Day 1:

Breakfast	Muesli (page 115)
Snack	Cranberry Cinnamon Bran Muffin (page 240)
Lunch	Mushroom Barley and Beef Soup (page 138)
	Open-face turkey sandwich with Sage and
	Tomato White Bean Dip (page 234)
	Carrot and celery sticks
Snack	Orange and fat- and sugar-free
	fruit-flavoured yogurt
Dinner	Hunter-Style Chicken (page 199)
	Long-grain rice and asparagus
Snack	Basmati Rice Pudding (page 248)

Day 2:

Breakfast	Homey Oatmeal (page 117)
	Grapefruit sections with 1% cottage cheese
Snack	Cranberry Cinnamon Bran Muffin (page 240)
Lunch	Tuscan White Bean Soup (page 133)
	Barbecue Chicken Salad (page 158)
	Whole wheat pita half
Snack	Apple and 1% cottage cheese
Dinner	Almond Haddock Fillets (page 182)
	Baby carrots and long-grain rice
	Zucchini Salad (page 147)
Snack	Apple Pie Cookie (page 253)

Day 3:

Breakfast	Back Bacon Omelette (page 125)
	Slice of 100% stone-ground whole wheat toast
	Tomato wedges
Snack	Whole Wheat Scone (page 238)

Lunch	Lemon Dill Lentil Salad (page 154)
	Open-face ham sandwich with Roasted Red Pepper Hummus (page 236)
	Pickle
Snack	Apple Pie Cookie (page 253) and glass of skim milk
Dinner	Asian Greens and Tofu Stir-fry (page 176)
	Basmati rice
	Tossed salad
Snack	Fresh Fruit Bowl (page 235)

Day 4:

Breakfast	Muesli (page 115)
	Back bacon
	Slice of 100% stone-ground whole wheat toast
	Sliced peach
Snack	Whole Wheat Scone (page 238)
Lunch	Ham and Lentil Soup (page 137)
	Tangy Red and Green Coleslaw (page 146)
	Whole wheat pita half
Snack	Baby carrots, broccoli and cucumber with Roasted Red Pepper Hummus (page 236)
Dinner	Horseradish Burger (page 208)
	Mediterranean Bean Salad (page 152)
Snack	Pecan Brownie (page 254) and glass of skim milk

Day 5:

Breakfast	Cinnamon French Toast (page 120)
	Sliced ham
	Orange
Snack	Almond Bran Haystack (page 252) and glass of skim milk
Lunch	Crab Salad in Tomato Shells (page 160)
	Cottage cheese with applesauce
Snack	Peach and fat- and sugar-free fruit-flavoured yogurt

Dinner   Veal with Fennel and Mushrooms (page 222)
           Spaghetti
           Steamed baby carrots
           Tomato Zucchini Wheat Berry Salad (page 156)
Snack   Berry Crumble (page 249)

Day 6:

Breakfast Puffy Baked Apple Omelette (page 124)
           Back bacon
Snack   Almond Bran Haystack (page 252) and a glass of
           skim milk
Lunch   Pepper and Tomato Beef Salad (page 162)
Snack   Tofu pudding
Dinner   Easy Bake Lasagna (page 178)
           Tossed salad
Snack   Poached Pears (page 247) with
           sweetened Yogurt Cheese (page 114)

Day 7:

Breakfast Morning Glory Poached Fruit (page 116)
           Florentine Frittata (page 126)
           Slice of 100% stone-ground whole wheat toast
Snack   Fat- and sugar-free fruit-flavoured yogurt
Lunch   Avocado and Fresh Fruit Salad (page 151)
           Open-face chicken sandwich with Roasted Red
           Pepper Hummus (page 236)
Snack   Dried Chickpeas (page 233)
Dinner   Salmon Steaks with Light Dill Tartar Sauce (page 185)
           Green beans and new potatoes
           Creamy Cucumber Salad (page 143)
Snack   Glazed Apple Tart (page 250)

CHAPTER TEN

The Recipes

Breakfast

Yogurt Smoothies

You don't need an expensive appliance to make these fruit-flavoured smoothies—a simple whisk will do.

2 cups	skim milk
1	container (175 g) non-fat sugar-free fruit-flavoured yogurt
½ tsp	sugar substitute

—

1. In tall glass or small bowl, whisk together milk, yogurt and sugar substitute until smooth.

Makes 2 servings.

—

Options

Thicker Smoothies: Break out the blender and add 1 cup sliced strawberries or raspberries.

Dessert Smoothies: Use 1 cup low-fat, no-added-sugar ice cream instead of the yogurt and buzz up with the milk, omitting sugar substitute.

Yogurt Cheese

This can be used as a tasty spread for whole wheat toast in the morning, as a dip, or as a topping for a dessert. Yogurt cheese is also a great substitute for sour cream in most recipes.

1 tub (750 g) plain low-fat yogurt

—

1. Dump tub of yogurt into cheesecloth-lined or clean tea towel–lined sieve. Place over large bowl. Cover with plastic wrap and refrigerate for at least 4 hours or overnight. Discard liquid and place yogurt cheese in airtight container.

Makes 1½ cups.

—

Options

Sweet Yogurt Cheese: You can sweeten your yogurt cheese by adding some sugar substitute to taste.

Lemony Yogurt Cheese: Add 1 tsp grated lemon rind and 2 tsp lemon juice along with sugar substitute to taste.

Quick Yogurt Cheese Dip: Simply add 2 green onions, chopped; 1 small clove garlic, minced; 1 tbsp lemon juice; and 1 tbsp chopped fresh oregano (or 1 tsp dried) to the yogurt cheese.

Helpful Hint: Be sure to keep the container the yogurt came in and write down the best-before date—that's how long your yogurt cheese is good for.

Muesli   GREEN-LIGHT

My friend Lesleigh introduced me to this delicious and healthy start to the day. Be sure to prepare it the night before so that it's ready to enjoy in the morning. Combine ⅓ cup of the Muesli with ⅓ cup of skim milk or water, and cover and refrigerate overnight. Then in the morning, combine the mixture with 1 container (175 g) of non-fat, sugar-free fruit yogurt and enjoy it cold, or pop it in the microwave for a hot breakfast.

2 cups	large-flake oats
¾ cup	oat bran
¾ cup	sliced almonds
½ cup	shelled unsalted sunflower seeds
2 tbsp	wheat germ
¼ tsp	cinnamon

1. In large resealable plastic bag, combine oats, oat bran, almonds, sunflower seeds, wheat germ and cinnamon. Using rolling pin, crush mixture into coarse crumbs. Shake bag to combine mixture.

Makes 3½ cups.

Storage: Keep in resealable bag or airtight container at room temperature for up to 1 month.

Morning Glory Poached Fruit   GREEN-LIGHT

*If you don't have time to eat breakfast at home, make this fruit the
night before or a few days before and take it with you. It also makes
a wonderful mid-morning or mid-afternoon snack.*

2	apples, cored and coarsely chopped
2	pears, cored and coarsely chopped
1	grapefruit
1	orange
2 cups	1% cottage cheese or Yogurt Cheese (see recipe on page 114)

Cinnamon Syrup:

2 cups	water
2	cinnamon sticks, broken in half
4	slices fresh ginger
3 tbsp	sugar substitute

—

1. Cinnamon Syrup: In small pot, bring water, cinnamon sticks,
ginger and sugar substitute to boil. Reduce heat to simmer and
add apples and pears. Cook for about 5 minutes or until tender-
crisp. Remove fruit with slotted spoon to large bowl, reserving
syrup. Let cool.

2. Meanwhile, using serrated knife, cut both ends of grapefruit off.
Starting at one end, cut skin and white pith off grapefruit, leaving
fruit intact. Repeat with orange. Using same knife, cut segments
between membranes of grapefruit and orange and add, along
with juices, to bowl with apples and pears. Serve with cottage
cheese and drizzle with some of the Cinnamon Syrup, if desired.

Makes 4 servings.

Storage: You can make this mixture up to 3 days ahead. Store in
an airtight container in the refrigerator.

Homey Oatmeal

This hot breakfast is guaranteed to keep you feeling satisfied all morning. You can vary the flavour by topping it with fresh fruit such as berries or chopped apple.

2 cups	skim milk
1 ½ cups	water
¾ tsp	cinnamon
½ tsp	salt
1⅓ cups	large-flake oats
¼ cup	wheat germ
¼ cup	chopped almonds
3 tbsp	sugar substitute

—

1. In large pot, bring milk, water, cinnamon and salt to boil. Stir in oats and wheat germ and return to boil. Reduce heat to low and cook, stirring, for about 8 minutes or until thickened. Stir in almonds and sugar substitute.

Makes 4 servings.

—

Wheat Berry Breakfast

This recipe comes from G.I. dieter Gwyneth, who has been making it for many years—especially during canoe trips. You can buy wheat berries, also known as soft or hard wheat kernels, at health or bulk food stores. Letting them sit overnight allows them to crack open, producing a delicate kernel of wheat.

1 cup	wheat berries
4 cups	water
	Skim milk
	Sugar substitute
	Sliced almonds
	Fresh fruit (such as berries or peaches)

—

1. In pot, add wheat berries and water; bring to boil. Reduce heat and simmer for 20 minutes.

2. Place wheat berries and water into large Thermos, Mason jar or heatproof airtight container and seal tightly. Let stand overnight.

3. Drain any water from wheat berries. Serve about ¾ cup of them with milk, sugar substitute, almonds and fruit as desired.

Makes about 3 servings.

—

Helpful Hint: If there are any leftovers, be sure to refrigerate them.

Buttermilk Pancakes   GREEN-LIGHT

This recipe comes from Michelle R. Though buttermilk may sound as though it's rich and indulgent, it's actually low fat and adds a wonderful tang to these pancakes.

2 cups	whole wheat flour
1 tbsp	baking powder
2 tsp	sugar substitute
2 cups	buttermilk
⅓ cup	liquid egg
2 tbsp	canola oil
1 ½ tsp	vanilla

—

1. In large bowl, combine whole wheat flour, baking powder and sugar substitute. In another bowl, whisk together buttermilk, liquid egg, canola oil and vanilla. Pour buttermilk mixture over flour mixture and whisk until smooth.

2. Heat non-stick griddle or large non-stick skillet over medium heat. Ladle batter onto griddle. Cook for about 2 minutes or until bubbles appear on top. Using spatula, flip pancake and cook for another minute or until golden. Repeat with remaining batter.

Makes about 16 pancakes, enough for 4 to 6 servings.

—

Cinnamon French Toast

Serve this family favourite with slices of ham or back bacon and extra strawberries for a complete breakfast.

¾ cup	liquid egg
½ cup	skim milk
1 tbsp	sugar substitute
1 tsp	vanilla
½ tsp	cinnamon
Pinch	salt
4	slices stone-ground whole wheat bread
1 tsp	canola oil
2 cups	sliced strawberries
½ cup	non-fat sugar-free fruit-flavoured yogurt

—

1. In shallow dish, whisk together liquid egg, milk, sugar substitute, vanilla, cinnamon and salt. Dip each slice of bread into egg mixture, making sure to coat both sides.

2. Meanwhile, brush oil onto non-stick griddle or large non-stick skillet over medium-high heat. Cook bread for about 4 minutes, turning once, or until golden brown. Serve each slice with strawberries and yogurt.

Makes 2 servings.

—

Light 'n' Fluffy Pancakes   GREEN-LIGHT

Pancakes make weekend mornings special. You can also enjoy them during the work week by making and freezing them ahead of time. When Tuesday or Wednesday rolls around, simply pop the frozen pancakes into your toaster or microwave and enjoy.

1¼ cups	all-purpose flour
¾ cup	whole wheat flour
¼ cup	wheat bran
1 tbsp	baking powder
¼ tsp	salt
¼ tsp	nutmeg
1½ cups	skim milk
½ cup	liquid egg
2 tbsp	canola oil
2 tbsp	sugar substitute
1 tsp	vanilla

—

1. In large bowl, combine all-purpose and whole wheat flours, bran, baking powder, salt and nutmeg. In another bowl, whisk together milk, liquid egg, oil, sugar substitute and vanilla. Pour milk mixture over flour mixture and whisk until smooth.

2. Heat non-stick griddle or large non-stick skillet over medium heat. Ladle batter onto griddle. Cook for about 2 minutes or until bubbles appear on top. Using spatula, flip pancake and cook for another minute or until golden. Repeat with remaining batter.

Makes about 16 pancakes, enough for 4 to 6 servings.

—

Storage: These pancakes can be frozen in a single layer on a baking sheet until firm. Place them in an airtight container once frozen.

Berry Crepes

GREEN-LIGHT

Crepes may sound difficult to make, but they are actually quite simple. Just make sure the pan is hot when you add the crepe batter. It should start to set as soon as you swirl it around the pan.

½ cup	whole wheat flour
1 tbsp	ground flax seed or wheat germ
Pinch	salt
1 cup	skim milk
½ cup	liquid egg
1 tsp	vanilla
1 tsp	canola oil
2 cups	each fresh blueberries and raspberries
2 tbsp	sugar substitute
1 tbsp	chopped fresh mint (optional)
Pinch	cinnamon
1 cup	Yogurt Cheese (see recipe page 114)

—

1. In bowl, combine flour, flax seed and salt. In another bowl, whisk together milk, liquid egg and vanilla. Pour over flour mixture and whisk until smooth. Let stand at room temperature for at least 15 minutes, or cover and refrigerate mixture for up to 2 hours.

2. Heat small non-stick or crepe pan over medium heat; brush with some of the oil. Pour in scant ¼ cup of the batter, swirling pan to cover bottom. Cook for about 2 minutes or until firm and slightly golden. Turn and cook other side for another 30 seconds. Remove to plate and repeat with remaining batter.

3. In large bowl, combine blueberries, raspberries, sugar substitute, mint (if using) and cinnamon. Put about ⅓ cup of the berry mixture in the centre of each crepe and roll up. Serve with Yogurt Cheese and remaining berries.

Makes about 10 crepes, enough for 4 servings.

—

Note: Sometimes the first crepe doesn't work out, so the recipe gives you a bit of extra batter to practise. If you're a pro at it, you'll have another serving of crepes.

Puffy Baked Apple Omelette GREEN-LIGHT

You can replace the apple in this recipe with your favourite seasonal fruit. Try peaches or pears.

4	cooking apples, cored
2 tsp	non-hydrogenated soft margarine
1/3 cup	apple juice
1/4 tsp	nutmeg
Pinch	each allspice and cloves
1 3/4 cups	liquid egg
1/2 cup	skim milk
1/2 cup	large-flake oats
1/4 cup	whole wheat flour
1/4 tsp	salt

—

1. Cut each apple into 8 slices. Meanwhile, in large non-stick skillet over medium heat, heat margarine; add apple slices, apple juice, nutmeg, allspice and cloves. Cook for about 15 minutes or until tender-crisp. Place apple slices into 8-inch square baking dish; set aside.

2. In large bowl, whisk together liquid egg, milk, oats, flour and salt. Pour over apples and bake in 350°F oven for about 20 minutes or until puffed and golden brown and knife inserted in centre comes out clean.

Makes 4 servings.

—

Speedy Option: Substitute a large can of sliced peaches or pears in water, drained, for the apples—no cooking required.

Back Bacon Omelette   GREEN-LIGHT

The smoky flavour of bacon makes this omelette a hit. Serve this with fresh fruit and yogurt for a hearty breakfast.

1 tsp	canola oil
½ cup	liquid egg
1 tbsp	chopped fresh basil or ½ tsp dried
1 tbsp	grated Parmesan cheese
Pinch	pepper
2	slices back bacon or ham, chopped
Quarter	red or green bell pepper, chopped

—

1. In small non-stick skillet, heat oil over medium-high heat. In bowl, using fork, stir together liquid egg, basil, cheese and pepper. Pour into skillet and cook for about 5 minutes, lifting edges to allow uncooked eggs to run underneath, until almost set.

2. Add bacon and red or green pepper over half of the omelette. Using spatula, fold over other half and cook for 1 minute. Slide onto plate.

Makes 1 serving.

—

Filling Options: Try other fillings for your omelette, like ½ cup chopped cooked spinach or Swiss chard or asparagus or ¼ cup light-style Swiss or havarti cheese. For seafood lovers, try ½ cup baby shrimp or crabmeat.

Florentine Frittata

A frittata is an easy Italian omelette that doesn't require flipping. You just pop it under the broiler to finish it off. It also makes a delicious lunch served on a slice of stone-ground whole wheat toast with a side of tossed salad.

2 tsp	extra-virgin olive oil
1	small onion, diced
2	cloves garlic, minced
1	red bell pepper, chopped
2 tbsp	chopped fresh oregano or 2 tsp dried
1	bag (300 g) fresh baby spinach
½ tsp	salt
1¼ cups	liquid egg
¼ cup	skim milk
Pinch	pepper

1. In large non-stick skillet with ovenproof handle, heat oil over medium-high heat; add onion, garlic, red pepper and oregano. Cook, stirring, for about 5 minutes or until golden. Add spinach and half of the salt; cover and cook for about 2 minutes or until spinach is wilted.

2. In bowl, whisk together liquid egg, skim milk, remaining salt and pepper. Pour into skillet, stirring gently to combine with spinach mixture. Cook, stirring gently, for about 2 minutes, lifting edges to allow uncooked egg to run underneath. Cook for another 3 minutes or until top is set. Place skillet under broiler for about 3 minutes or until golden brown and knife inserted in centre comes out clean.

Makes 2 servings.

Shrimp and
Mushroom Omelette

GREEN-LIGHT

This omelette is a hit with my husband on weekend mornings.
It would also make a special addition to any brunch table.

8 oz	small raw shrimp, peeled and deveined
4 tsp	canola oil
Half	small onion, diced
2	cloves garlic, minced
2 cups	sliced mushrooms
2 tsp	chopped fresh thyme leaves or ½ tsp dried
¼ tsp	salt
Pinch	pepper
Half	red bell pepper, halved and thinly sliced
1¼ cups	liquid egg
⅓ cup	chopped fresh Italian parsley

—

1. In large non-stick skillet, heat 1 tsp of the oil over medium-high heat; cook shrimp for about 4 minutes or until pink. Remove to bowl and keep warm. Return skillet to medium-high heat and add 1 tsp of the oil. Cook onion and garlic for about 2 minutes or until starting to brown. Add mushrooms, thyme, salt and pepper; cook, stirring, for about 8 minutes or until all liquid is evaporated and mushrooms are golden. Stir in red pepper and add mixture to cooked shrimp.

2. In same skillet, heat remaining oil over medium heat. In bowl, using fork, stir together liquid egg and parsley. Pour into skillet and cook for about 5 minutes, lifting edges to allow uncooked egg to run underneath, or until set.

3. Add shrimp and mushroom mixture over half of the omelette. Using spatula, fold over other half and cook for 1 minute. Slide onto plate and cut in half.

Makes 2 servings.

—

Soups

Navy Bean Soup GREEN-LIGHT

This recipe comes from Beth F., who went on the G.I. Diet after hearing about it on a local radio show. She and her husband are both enjoying the new way of eating and like having this thick and nourishing soup for lunch.

12 cups	water
2 cups	dry navy beans
2	carrots, chopped
1	large onion, chopped
1	celery stalk, chopped
1	bay leaf
1 tsp	salt
Pinch	pepper
	Tabasco sauce

—

1. In soup pot, bring 8 cups of the water and beans to boil. Reduce heat and simmer for about 1 hour or until beans are almost tender. Add remaining water, carrots, onion, celery and bay leaf and cook for about 1 hour or until vegetables and beans are tender. Remove bay leaf. Add salt and pepper. Serve with Tabasco, if desired.

Makes 4 servings.

—

Hearty Onion Soup   GREEN-LIGHT

I don't make this yummy soup often enough. If you don't have French onion soup bowls, you can ladle the soup into microwave-safe bowls and melt the cheese in the microwave. Add a splash of Tabasco sauce for an added kick.

1 tbsp	canola oil
6	onions, thinly sliced
2	cloves garlic, minced
½ tsp	salt
2 tbsp	whole wheat flour
6 cups	beef stock (low fat, low sodium)
½ cup	red wine
2 tbsp	dry sherry or cognac
1	bay leaf
½ tsp	pepper
4	slices stone-ground whole wheat toasts
1 cup	shredded light-style Swiss or Jarlsberg cheese

1. In soup pot, heat oil over medium-high heat. Cook onions, garlic and salt, stirring often, for about 10 minutes or until they start to brown. Reduce heat to medium-low and continue cooking, stirring occasionally, for about 20 minutes or until onions are very golden and very soft. Add flour and stir to coat onions for 1 minute.

2. Add beef stock, wine, sherry, bay leaf and pepper; bring to boil. Reduce heat and simmer for 30 minutes. Remove bay leaf.

3. Pour soup into desired bowls. Place bread on top to fit bowls and sprinkle with cheese. Bake in 400°F oven for about 15 minutes or until cheese is bubbly. Broil for 30 seconds to brown top.

Makes 4 servings.

Lighter Option: For an even lighter soup, omit cheese and bread.

Storage: You can make this soup through to step 2 up to 3 days ahead. Let cool to room temperature in pot; cover and refrigerate. Reheat before continuing with step 3.

Helpful Hint: To make your own toasts, place bread slices on baking sheet. Bake in 350°F oven for about 20 minutes, turning once, or until dried.

Miso Soup

This is a great starter for an Asian-inspired dinner. Miso is fermented soybean paste that ranges in colour from white to dark brown. The lighter the colour, the milder the flavour. Since miso tends to sink to the bottom, be sure to stir up your soup as you eat it to get its full rich flavour.

4 cups	vegetable stock (low fat, low sodium)
2 cups	water
1	sheet nori
1 cup	diced firm tofu
1 cup	sliced mushrooms
3	green onions, chopped
3 tbsp	miso paste
1 tbsp	soy sauce

—

1. In soup pot, bring stock and water to boil.

2. Meanwhile, tear nori into small bite-size pieces. Add nori, tofu, mushrooms, green onions, miso and soy sauce to pot. Reduce heat and simmer for about 20 minutes or until nori and mushrooms are tender.

Makes 4 servings.

—

Helpful Hints: Nori is used to make sushi rolls in Japanese cooking. Look for nori, also known as toasted seaweed, in the International section of your grocery store. Some grocery stores sell sushi and will have the ingredients to sell as well. Or check your local Asian grocery.

You can find miso in health and bulk food stores as well as in Asian groceries and some specialty food shops.

Tuscan White Bean Soup   GREEN-LIGHT

I first tried this country-style soup in Tuscany and immediately fell in love with it. I serve this soup in deep Italian ceramic soup bowls and dream I'm back in Tuscany.

1 tbsp	extra-virgin olive oil
1	onion, chopped
4	cloves garlic, minced
1	carrot, chopped
1	celery stalk, chopped
4	fresh sage leaves or ½ tsp dried
6 cups	vegetable or chicken stock (low fat, low sodium)
2	cans (540 ml) cannellini or white kidney beans, drained and rinsed
4 cups	shredded kale
Pinch	each salt and pepper

—

1. In soup pot, heat oil over medium heat. Add onion, garlic, carrot, celery and sage and cook for 5 minutes or until softened.

2. Add stock, beans, kale, salt and pepper, and cook, stirring occasionally, for about 20 minutes or until kale is tender.

Makes 4 servings.

—

Minestrone Soup

This soup is one of my favourites because it contains both pasta and spinach. Serve it with a sprinkling of grated Parmesan for extra flavour and a few more red pepper flakes to get your blood pumping.

2 tsp	canola oil
3	slices back bacon, chopped
1	onion, chopped
4	cloves garlic, minced
2	carrots, chopped
1	celery stalk, chopped
1 tbsp	dried oregano
½ tsp	red pepper flakes
¼ tsp	each salt and pepper
1	can (796 ml) plum tomatoes
6 cups	chicken stock (low fat, low sodium)
1	bag (300 g) baby spinach
1	can (540 ml) each red kidney beans and chickpeas, drained and rinsed
¾ cup	ditali or tubetti pasta
⅓ cup	chopped fresh Italian parsley
2 tbsp	chopped fresh basil (optional)

—

1. In soup pot, heat oil over medium-high heat and cook back bacon for 2 minutes. Reduce heat to medium and add onion, garlic, carrots, celery, oregano, red pepper flakes, salt and pepper. Cook for about 10 minutes or until softened and just about golden.

2. Add tomatoes and crush using potato masher in pot. Pour in chicken stock; bring to boil. Reduce heat to simmer and add spinach, beans, chickpeas and pasta. Simmer for about 20 minutes or until pasta is tender. Stir in parsley and basil (if using).

Makes 6 servings.

—

Vegetarian Option: Omit back bacon and use vegetable stock for the chicken stock.

Smoky Black Bean Soup   GREEN-LIGHT

Whenever I make this soup, my husband always asks for more. The wonderful flavour of smoked turkey permeates it. Look for smoked turkey legs in the deli section of your grocery store.

1 tbsp	canola oil
1	onion, diced
2	cloves garlic, minced
1	jalapeno pepper, seeded and minced
2	cans (540 ml each) black beans, drained and rinsed
6 cups	chicken stock (low fat, low sodium)
1	smoked turkey leg (about 1¼ lb)
¼ cup	tomato paste
2	green bell peppers, diced
1	tomato, seeded and diced
⅓ cup	chopped fresh coriander
¼ cup	light sour cream

—

1. In soup pot, heat oil over medium heat. Cook onion, garlic and jalapeno pepper for about 3 minutes or until softened. Add beans, stock, turkey leg and tomato paste. Bring to boil; reduce heat and simmer for about 1 hour or until turkey begins to break apart.

2. Remove turkey leg and set aside. Pour soup into blender in batches and purée until smooth. Return to pot over medium heat. Add peppers and tomato and heat until steaming.

3. Meanwhile, remove meat from turkey leg and chop; add to soup. Serve sprinkled with coriander and a dollop of sour cream.

Makes 4 servings.

—

Ham Option: You can substitute smoked ham or hamhock for the turkey leg.

Ham and Lentil Soup

GREEN-LIGHT

Canned lentils make this soup quick and easy to prepare, so keep some on hand in the pantry. If you want to make this soup even more green-light, use dried lentils (see instructions at the bottom of this page).

1 tbsp	canola oil
1	onion, chopped
½ cup	diced celery
2	cloves garlic, minced
6 cups	chicken stock (low fat, low sodium)
2	cans (540 ml each) lentils, drained and rinsed
6 oz	black forest ham, diced
1	red bell pepper, diced
2	tomatoes, seeded and diced
2 tbsp	chopped fresh Italian parsley

—

1. In soup pot, heat oil over medium heat and cook onion, celery and garlic for about 5 minutes or until softened. Add stock, lentils, ham and red pepper; bring to boil. Reduce heat and add tomatoes. Cover and simmer for 20 minutes. Stir in parsley.

Makes 4 servings.

—

Dried Lentil Option: Use 1 cup dried green or brown lentils. Add with stock, and cover and simmer for about 30 minutes or until tender.

Mushroom Barley and Beef Soup

GREEN-LIGHT

A thick, hearty stew-like soup will warm up anyone on a cold winter's night. This is real comfort food for the soul and the belly.

1 tbsp	canola oil
8 oz	extra-lean ground beef
1	onion, chopped
2	cloves garlic, minced
1 lb	mushrooms, sliced
1	each carrot and celery stalk, chopped
1 tbsp	chopped fresh thyme leaves or 1 tsp dried
2 tbsp	tomato paste
1 tbsp	balsamic vinegar
¼ tsp	each salt and pepper
4 cups	beef stock (low fat, low sodium)
3 cups	water
½ cup	barley
1	bay leaf
1	can (540 ml) black beans, drained and rinsed

—

1. In large deep pot, heat oil over medium-high heat and cook beef until no longer pink. Reduce heat to medium and add onion and garlic; cook, stirring, for 5 minutes. Add mushrooms, carrot, celery and thyme and cook for about 15 minutes or until all liquid has evaporated from mushrooms.

2. Add tomato paste, vinegar, salt and pepper; stir to coat vegetables. Add stock, water, barley and bay leaf; bring to boil. Reduce heat, cover and simmer for about 45 minutes or until barley is tender. Add beans and heat through. Remove bay leaf.

Makes 4 to 6 servings.

—

Chicken Option: You can use ground chicken or turkey for the beef and use chicken stock instead of beef stock.

Note: Mushrooms come in all shapes and sizes. The best for this soup are your favourites: white or brown (cremini) mushrooms, shiitakes, oyster mushrooms or even portobellos.

Cioppino

This Italian-influenced fish stew can be made with whatever happens to be the fresh catch of the day. Adding shellfish such as crab, clams or lobster will make it impressive enough for entertaining.

1 tbsp	olive oil
1	onion, chopped
4	cloves garlic, minced
1	green bell pepper, chopped
1	can (796 ml) diced tomatoes, drained
1 cup	fish or chicken stock (low fat, low sodium)
½ cup	red wine
½ cup	chopped fresh Italian parsley
1 tsp	dried oregano
½ tsp	dried basil or 2 tbsp chopped fresh
½ tsp	red pepper flakes
½ lb	mussels, rinsed
½ lb	cod fillets
½ lb	large, raw shrimp, peeled and deveined

—

1. In soup pot, heat oil over medium heat. Cook onion, garlic and pepper for about 5 minutes or until softened. Add tomatoes, fish stock, wine, ¼ cup of the parsley, oregano, basil and red pepper flakes; bring to boil. Reduce heat and simmer for 15 minutes.

2. Meanwhile scrub mussels and remove beards; discard any mussels that do not close when tapped. Add mussels, cod and shrimp to pot; cover and cook for about 5 minutes or until mussels are open and cod and shrimp are firm. Gently stir in remaining ¼ cup of parsley.

Makes 3 servings.

—

Thai Shrimp Soup

This soup is a huge favourite of my sister's. You can make it with chicken or scallops instead of the shrimp. Look for lemongrass in the fresh herb section of the produce aisle in the grocery store. Cut the top grassy part off and use the thicker bottom part. Hit the stalk with the back of your knife to release some of the juices before cutting. If you can't find lemongrass, use 4 large strips of lemon rind instead.

4 cups	chicken or vegetable stock (low fat, low sodium)
¼ cup	thinly sliced fresh ginger
2	lemongrass stalks, cut in 1-inch pieces
1	clove garlic, minced
1 tbsp	minced hot pepper or ¼ tsp red pepper flakes
1 lb	large raw shrimp, peeled and deveined
4 oz	rice vermicelli noodles
2 cups	bean sprouts
2	green onions, chopped
2 tbsp	rice vinegar
¼ cup	fresh coriander leaves

—

1. In soup pot, bring stock, ginger, lemongrass, garlic and hot pepper to boil. Reduce heat and simmer for 15 minutes. Add shrimp, noodles, sprouts and green onions; cook, stirring, for about 5 minutes or until shrimp are pink and noodles are tender.

2. Serve each bowlful with splash of vinegar and sprinkle of coriander.

Makes 4 to 6 servings.

—

Note: Ginger and lemongrass are both too tough to eat but provide plenty of flavour.

Salads

Creamy Cucumber Salad GREEN-LIGHT

This salad is reminiscent of veggies and dip. Use an English cucumber if available, but if not, use a field cucumber and remove the seeds.

1	cucumber
2 cups	grape tomatoes, halved
⅓ cup	light sour cream
⅓ cup	light mayonnaise
2 tbsp	chopped fresh dill or 2 tsp dried
1	small clove garlic, minced
½ tsp	grated lemon rind
1 tbsp	lemon juice
½ tsp	each salt and pepper
¼ tsp	celery seed, crushed

1. Cut off ends of cucumber. Cut in half lengthwise; cut into thin slices. Place in large bowl with tomatoes and set aside.

2. In small bowl, whisk together sour cream, mayonnaise, dill, garlic, lemon rind and juice, salt, pepper and celery seed. Pour over cucumber mixture and stir gently to coat.

Makes 4 servings.

Options: This salad is delicious combined with bell peppers, carrots, radishes, broccoli or cauliflower instead of tomatoes.

Bacon Spinach Salad
with Buttermilk Dressing   GREEN-LIGHT

The classic combination of bacon and spinach is always a surefire hit. If you plan to take this salad with you for lunch, pack up the greens and dressing separately.

6	slices back bacon
1	bag (300 g) fresh baby spinach
1 cup	cooked chickpeas
4	radishes, thinly sliced
1 cup	bean sprouts
1	red bell pepper, thinly sliced
⅓ cup	thinly sliced red onion

Creamy Buttermilk Dressing:

¼ cup	buttermilk or light sour cream
2 tbsp	light mayonnaise
1 tbsp	cider vinegar
2 tsp	poppy seeds
1 tsp	Dijon mustard
½ tsp	sugar substitute
¼ tsp	each salt and pepper

—

1. In non-stick skillet, cook back bacon over medium-high heat until crisp. Let cool and chop coarsely. In large bowl, toss together spinach, chickpeas, radishes, bean sprouts, red pepper and onion.

2. Creamy Buttermilk Dressing: In small bowl, whisk together buttermilk, mayonnaise, vinegar, poppy seeds, mustard, sugar substitute, salt and pepper.

3. Pour dressing over salad and toss gently to coat. Sprinkle with back bacon and toss again.

Makes 4 servings.

—

Make ahead: You can make the dressing up to 3 days ahead and store it in the refrigerator. You can also prepare the salad greens up to 1 day ahead.

Orange Salad Option: Omit bacon from recipe. Cut rind and pith from 2 oranges and slice fruit into thin rounds; add to spinach. Orange Dressing: Omit buttermilk and add ¼ cup orange juice.

Tangy Red and Green Coleslaw

GREEN-LIGHT

Using a vinaigrette in coleslaw makes it low fat and really tangy! This is a great keeper salad for the refrigerator or to tote along to a potluck.

4 cups	finely shredded green cabbage
2 cups	finely shredded red cabbage
2	carrots, shredded
½ cup	thinly sliced celery
¼ cup	chopped fresh Italian parsley
½ cup	cider vinegar
2 tbsp	canola oil
2 tsp	sugar substitute
1 tsp	celery seeds
½ tsp	salt
Pinch	pepper

—

1. In large bowl, toss together green and red cabbage, carrots, celery and parsley.

2. In small bowl, whisk together vinegar, oil, sugar substitute, celery seeds, salt and pepper. Pour over cabbage mixture and toss to coat.

Makes 4 to 6 servings.

—

Storage: Cover and refrigerate for up to 2 days.

Creamy Coleslaw Dressing Option: Whisk together ¼ cup each plain yogurt and light mayonnaise, 2 tbsp cider vinegar, 1 tbsp Dijon mustard, 2 tsp sugar substitute, ½ tsp celery seed and ¼ tsp salt.

Zucchini Salad

Here's a new way to use up the zucchini that may be overrunning your garden. Serve this crunchy salad as a side dish with Grilled Rosemary Chicken Thighs (see recipe page 197).

6	zucchini, trimmed
2	red bell peppers, chopped
¼ cup	chopped fresh Italian parsley
¼ cup	chopped fresh basil
3 tbsp	balsamic vinegar
2 tbsp	extra-virgin olive oil
2	cloves garlic, minced
¼ tsp	each salt and pepper
4 oz	sliced prosciutto, fat removed

—

1. Cut zucchini in half lengthwise; cut into ½-inch thick slices. In large pot of boiling water, blanch zucchini for 1 minute or until bright green and tender-crisp. Drain and plunge zucchini into cold ice water to chill and stop the cooking process. Drain again, shaking off excess water; set aside.

2. In large bowl, toss together blanched zucchini, peppers, parsley and basil. In small bowl, whisk together vinegar, oil, garlic, salt and pepper. Pour over zucchini; toss gently to coat.

3. Cut prosciutto into thin strips and sprinkle over salad.

Makes 4 to 6 servings.

—

Storage: Cover with plastic wrap and refrigerate for up to 1 day.

Ham Option: Substitute black forest ham, smoked turkey or cooked chicken for the prosciutto.

Arugula and Roasted Pepper Pasta Salad

GREEN-LIGHT

Peppery arugula is a perfect match for roasted sweet red peppers. Add some chopped cooked chicken, turkey or ham for lunch for the family. This salad will keep up to three days in the refrigerator.

3 cups	whole wheat fusilli or penne pasta
1	large bunch arugula, trimmed
1	jar (370 ml) roasted red peppers, drained
1	can (398 ml) artichokes, drained and chopped
4	green onions, chopped
2	tomatoes, seeded and chopped
¼ cup	white wine vinegar
2 tbsp	extra-virgin olive oil
1	small clove garlic, minced
1 tbsp	chopped fresh thyme or 1 tsp dried
2 tsp	Dijon mustard
¼ tsp	each salt and pepper

—

1. In large pot of boiling salted water, cook pasta for about 7 minutes or until al dente. Drain and rinse under cold water until pasta is cool; place in large bowl.

2. Tear arugula into bite-size pieces and add to pasta. Slice peppers into thin strips and add to pasta along with artichokes, green onions and tomatoes.

3. In small bowl, whisk together vinegar, oil, garlic, thyme, mustard, salt and pepper. Pour over salad and toss to coat.

Makes 4 to 6 servings.

—

Guacamole Salad

I've taken all the wonderful flavours of guacamole and put them into this delicious salad. Serve it as a starter for a Mexican-themed dinner, right before your Chicken Enchiladas or Beef Fajitas (see recipes on pages 204 and 210. Roll any leftovers in a whole wheat tortilla or stuff them into a pita for lunch the next day.

2	avocados, chopped
1	tomato, chopped
Half	yellow bell pepper, diced
⅓ cup	diced red onion
¼ tsp	grated lime rind
2 tbsp	lime juice
1 tbsp	canola oil
Pinch	salt
4 cups	shredded romaine lettuce
1	green onion, chopped

—

1. In large bowl, add avocado, tomato, pepper, onion, lime rind and juice, oil and salt. Toss gently to combine.

2. Divide lettuce onto 2 dinner plates. Top with avocado mixture; sprinkle with green onion.

Makes 4 servings.

—

Mozzarella and Tomato Stacks

This salad shows off the colours of the Italian flag and makes a great start to any Italian-themed meal. If fresh basil is unavailable, chop some Italian parsley and sprinkle it over the tomatoes and cheese.

3	small tomatoes, sliced
16	thin slices light mozzarella cheese
16	fresh basil leaves
2 tbsp	extra-virgin olive oil
2 tbsp	balsamic vinegar
1	clove garlic, minced
¼ tsp	pepper

—

1. Top each tomato slice with slice of cheese and basil leaf. Place stacks onto large platter.

2. In small bowl, whisk together oil, vinegar, garlic and pepper. Drizzle over cheese and tomato stacks.

Makes 4 servings.

—

Helpful Hint: Buy the small blocks (227 g) of mozzarella cheese to get perfect little cheese squares that fit nicely on the tomato slices.

Avocado and Fresh Fruit Salad   YELLOW-LIGHT

The avocado is a bit of a surprise in this refreshing salad, but it really does go well with fruit, providing a nice colour contrast and a rich creamy texture.

2 cups	torn red leaf lettuce
1	avocado, peeled and chopped
1	yellow bell pepper, chopped
Half	mango, peeled and chopped
Half	papaya, peeled and chopped
1	green onion, chopped
¼ cup	chopped fresh Italian parsley

Dijon Vinaigrette:

2 tbsp	canola oil
1 tsp	grated lime rind
1 tbsp	lime juice
1 tbsp	Dijon mustard
1	small clove garlic, minced
Pinch	dried thyme
Pinch	each salt and pepper

—

1. Dijon Vinaigrette: In small bowl, whisk together oil, lime rind and juice, mustard, garlic, thyme, salt and pepper; set aside.

2. In large bowl, toss together lettuce, avocado, pepper, mango, papaya, green onion and parsley. Pour vinaigrette over and toss.

Makes 2 servings.

—

Storage: To take this salad to work, simply pack up the vinaigrette separately from the salad and toss together once you're ready to eat.

Mediterranean Bean Salad

GREEN-LIGHT

This recipe is a fresh twist on classic bean salad. Bring it to the next potluck or pack it away for tomorrow's lunch.

8 oz	green beans, trimmed
¼ cup	sundried tomatoes
1	can (540 ml) chickpeas, drained and rinsed
1	can (540 ml) black beans, drained and rinsed
1	yellow or red bell pepper, diced
1 cup	diced sweet onion
3 tbsp	balsamic vinegar or lemon juice
1 tbsp	extra-virgin olive oil
½ tsp	each salt and pepper
½ cup	chopped mixed fresh herbs (such as parsley, mint and basil)

—

1. In pot of boiling salted water, blanch beans for 3 minutes. Drain and rinse under cold water; cut into 1-inch pieces. Place beans in large bowl; set aside.

2. Meanwhile, soak tomatoes in ½ cup of boiling water. Let stand for 10 minutes. Drain, reserving liquid. Chop tomatoes and add to beans. Add chickpeas, black beans, yellow pepper and onion.

3. In small bowl, whisk together vinegar, oil, 2 tbsp of the reserved liquid, and salt and pepper. Pour over salad and toss to coat. Add herbs and toss again.

Makes 4 to 6 servings.

—

Storage: Cover with plastic wrap and refrigerate for up to 2 days.

Bean Options: Use kidney, pinto or Romano beans for the chickpeas and black beans.

Corn Option: Add 1 can (398 ml) corn, drained, to salad for extra colour and flavour.

Lemon Dill Lentil Salad   GREEN-LIGHT

I really love the combination of lentils and chickpeas in this salad, but you can use other types of beans as well, such as red or white kidney beans. For another twist, add a sprinkle of feta cheese and a few olives.

1 tbsp	canola oil
1	onion, chopped
1	clove garlic, minced
1½ cups	water
½ cup	dried lentils
Pinch	pepper
1	can (540 ml) chickpeas, drained and rinsed
1	green bell pepper, chopped
1 cup	chopped cucumber
1 cup	halved grape tomatoes
½ cup	chopped fresh Italian parsley
4	lettuce leaves

Lemon Dill Dressing:

2 tbsp	canola oil
2 tbsp	chopped fresh dill or 1 tsp dried dillweed
½ tsp	grated lemon rind
1 tbsp	lemon juice
¼ tsp	each salt and pepper

———

1. In saucepan, heat oil over medium heat. Cook onion and garlic for 5 minutes or until softened. Add water, lentils and pepper; bring to boil. Reduce heat and simmer for 30 minutes or until lentils are tender. Let cool completely.

2. Meanwhile, in large bowl, combine chickpeas, green pepper, cucumber, tomatoes and parsley. Add cooled lentils.

3. Lemon Dill Dressing: In small bowl, whisk together oil, dill, lemon rind and juice, salt and pepper. Pour over salad and gently stir to coat. Serve salad on lettuce leaves.

Makes 4 servings.

—

Storage: Cover and refrigerate for up to 3 days.

Full-Meal Option: Add some cooked chicken, Black Forest ham or smoked turkey to this salad for a heartier meal.

Tomato Zucchini Wheat Berry Salad

GREEN-LIGHT

I love wheat berries because they have a wonderful nutty flavour and are very healthy. Cook up a large batch and put the extra in the freezer for another salad or a great addition to soups.

1 cup	wheat berries
1	zucchini, chopped
¼ cup	sundried tomatoes
2	plum tomatoes, chopped
¼ cup	chopped fresh basil
3 tbsp	balsamic vinegar
2 tsp	extra-virgin olive oil
1	clove garlic, minced
¼ tsp	salt
Pinch	pepper

1. In pot of boiling salted water, cook wheat berries, covered, for about 1 hour or until tender. Drain and rinse under cold water until cool. Place in bowl.

2. Meanwhile, in small pot of boiling water, blanch zucchini for 1 minute. Drain zucchini, reserving water, and rinse under cold water; add to wheat berries. Add sundried tomatoes to reserved water and let stand for 10 minutes or until softened. Drain and chop finely. Add to wheat berries with plum tomatoes and basil.

3. In small bowl, whisk together vinegar, oil, garlic, salt and pepper. Pour over wheat berry mixture and toss to coat.

Makes 4 servings.

—

Storage: Cover and refrigerate for up to 3 days.

Tabbouleh Salad

You often see this salad in the grocery store deli, but it's very simple to make at home. I've added chickpeas for more fibre. Use Italian parsley for the best flavour.

1½ cups	water
¾ cup	bulgur
½ tsp	grated lemon rind
2 tbsp	lemon juice
2 tbsp	extra-virgin olive oil
1	small clove garlic, minced
½ tsp	each salt and pepper
¼ tsp	ground cumin
1	can (540 ml) chickpeas, drained and rinsed
3	plum tomatoes, diced
Quarter	cucumber, diced
1 cup	finely chopped fresh Italian parsley
½ cup	finely chopped fresh mint
1 tbsp	chopped fresh chives

—

1. In saucepan, bring water to boil; add bulgur. Cover and reduce heat to low and cook for about 10 minutes or until water is absorbed. Using fork, scrape into large bowl; let cool.

2. In small bowl, whisk together lemon rind and juice, oil, garlic, salt, pepper and cumin; pour over bulgur. Stir in chickpeas, tomatoes, cucumber, parsley, mint and chives until well combined.

Makes 4 to 6 servings.

—

Storage: This salad will last up to 3 days in the refrigerator.

Barbecue Chicken Salad

You can add the chicken to this salad hot off the grill or barbecue it ahead of time and use it cold. For a totable lunch, stuff it into half of a whole wheat pita.

2 tbsp	soy sauce
2 tbsp	canola oil
2 tbsp	chopped fresh coriander
1 tbsp	minced fresh ginger
2	cloves garlic, minced
¼ tsp	Asian chili paste or red pepper flakes
4	boneless skinless chicken breasts
2	each red and yellow bell peppers
6 cups	mesclun greens
3 tbsp	rice vinegar
¼ tsp	salt

—

1. In large bowl, whisk together soy sauce, 1 tbsp of the canola oil, coriander, ginger, garlic and chili paste. Add chicken breasts and toss to coat well. Cover and refrigerate for at least 30 minutes or up to 1 day.

2. Meanwhile, cut peppers into quarters. Place on greased grill over medium-high heat. Grill for about 15 minutes, turning once, or until starting to blacken. Remove to plate. Place chicken breasts on greased grill over medium-high heat and grill for about 12 minutes, turning once, or until no longer pink inside. Remove to plate.

3. Chop grilled peppers and chicken into bite-size pieces. In large
   bowl, toss chicken and peppers with mesclun greens, remaining oil, vinegar and salt.

   Makes 4 servings.

   —

Storage: This salad will last up to 1 day in the refrigerator.

Roasting Option: You can roast the peppers and chicken instead
of barbecuing them. Place vegetables on parchment paper–lined
baking sheet and roast in 425°F oven for about 15 minutes. Add
chicken breasts and roast for another 12 minutes or until chicken
is no longer pink inside and peppers are blackened.

Crab Salad in Tomato Shells GREEN-LIGHT

Beefsteak tomatoes are ideal for this dish because their large size will accommodate the filling and because their pulp and seeds are easy to scoop out. Try using baby shrimp, tuna or salmon instead of the crab.

2	pkgs (each 200 g) frozen crab, thawed
4	large beefsteak tomatoes
¼ cup	light mayonnaise
2 tbsp	light sour cream
½ tsp	finely grated lemon rind
1 tbsp	lemon juice
2 tsp	chopped fresh tarragon or ½ tsp dried
Pinch	each salt and pepper
1 cup	coarsely chopped cooked chickpeas
Half	red bell pepper, diced
¼ cup	finely diced celery
¼ cup	chopped fresh Italian parsley
2 tbsp	chopped fresh chives
2 tbsp	shredded carrot

—

1. Place crab in fine mesh sieve; press out any liquid. Remove any cartilage if necessary and set aside.

2. Cut top quarter off tomatoes. Using small spoon, scoop out seeds and pulp. Place tomatoes cut-side down on paper towel–lined plate.

3. Meanwhile, in large bowl, whisk together mayonnaise, sour cream, lemon rind and juice, tarragon, salt and pepper. Add chickpeas, red bell pepper, celery, parsley, chives and carrot. Add crab and stir to combine. Divide crab mixture among tomatoes.

Makes 4 servings.

—

Herb Option: Substitute an additional 3 tbsp chopped fresh Italian parsley for chives and tarragon.

Seafood Option: Substitute 12 oz imitation crabmeat, chopped finely, or baby shrimp, or 2 cans (120 g each) tuna or salmon, for crabmeat.

Crab Melts: Omit tomatoes. Top 4 slices of stone-ground whole wheat bread with crab mixture and sprinkle with ½ cup of shredded light-style Swiss cheese. Place under broiler until melted. This makes a great lunch for 4 people.

Pepper and Tomato Beef Salad   GREEN-LIGHT

Thinly slicing the steak for this salad gives the illusion of a lot of meat while keeping everyone's serving size to the recommended 3 to 4 ounces.

2 tbsp	extra-virgin olive oil
2 tbsp	red wine vinegar
1 tsp	Worcestershire sauce
½ tsp	dried thyme leaves or 1 tbsp chopped fresh
½ tsp	salt
¼ tsp	pepper
8 oz	top sirloin grilling steak, 1 inch thick
3 cups	torn romaine lettuce or arugula
1	tomato, cut in wedges
Half	each red and green bell peppers, thinly sliced
Quarter	cucumber, thinly sliced
¼ cup	chopped fresh mint or parsley

—

1. In large shallow dish, whisk together 1 tbsp each of the oil and vinegar, Worcestershire sauce, thyme and a pinch each of the salt and pepper. Place steak in marinade and turn to coat. Cover and refrigerate for 30 minutes or up to 1 day.

2. Place steak on greased grill over medium-high heat and grill for 10 minutes, turning once, for medium-rare. Continue cooking steak to desired doneness. Remove to plate and tent with aluminum foil for 5 minutes.

3. Meanwhile, in large bowl, toss together lettuce, tomato, red and green peppers, cucumber and mint. Whisk together remaining oil, vinegar, salt and pepper. Drizzle over greens and toss to coat.

4. Slice steak into thin strips and add to salad. Toss to combine.

Makes 2 servings.

—

Chicken or Salmon Option: Substitute 2 boneless skinless chicken breasts or 2 salmon fillets for the steak.

Helpful Hint: To take this salad for lunch, simply pack the beef and salad separately. At lunchtime, add the two together.

Asian Grilled Tofu Salad GREEN-LIGHT

Marinating and grilling the tofu adds lots of flavour to this salad. Have it with a bowl of Miso Soup (see recipe page 132) for a terrific lunch.

1	pkg (350 g) extra-firm tofu
¼ cup	rice vinegar
3 tbsp	soy sauce
2 tbsp	chopped fresh coriander
1 tbsp	minced fresh ginger or ½ tsp dried
1	clove garlic, minced
¼ tsp	Asian chili paste or hot sauce
6 cups	mesclun greens
1 cup	grape tomatoes
½ cup	bean sprouts
2	green onions, chopped
2 tsp	canola oil

—

1. Cut tofu in half lengthwise into 2 pieces. Repeat with each piece to get 4 pieces of tofu; set aside.

2. In shallow glass dish, whisk together vinegar, soy sauce, coriander, ginger, garlic and chili paste. Add tofu to marinade, turning to coat. Cover and let stand for 30 minutes.

3. Meanwhile, in large bowl, toss together greens, tomatoes, bean sprouts and green onions; set aside.

4. Reserving marinade, grill tofu slices on greased grill over medium-high heat, turning once, for about 5 minutes, or until golden brown. Remove to cutting board and slice into thin strips. Pour ¼ cup of the remaining marinade and oil over greens and top with grilled tofu.

Makes 4 servings.

—

Storage: Cover and refrigerate marinated grilled tofu and greens separately for up to 1 day.

Grilled Shrimp Salad

The crisp clean flavour of mesclun complements the light spiciness of the shrimp in this salad. This dish is a good choice for entertaining friends for lunch. You can use arugula or baby spinach in it, too.

6 cups	mesclun greens
1 cup	sliced mushrooms
Half	red bell pepper, thinly sliced
1 tbsp	canola oil
2 tsp	mild curry paste or powder
2 tsp	lemon juice
1 tsp	grated fresh ginger
Pinch	salt
12 oz	jumbo raw shrimp, peeled and deveined

Orange Dressing:

1 tbsp	canola oil
½ tsp	grated orange rind
1 tbsp	orange juice
1 tbsp	lemon juice
1 tsp	Dijon mustard
1 tbsp	chopped fresh mint or ½ tsp dried
1	small clove garlic, minced
¼ tsp	salt

—

1. In large bowl, toss together greens, mushrooms and pepper; set aside.

2. Orange Dressing: In small bowl, whisk together oil, orange rind, orange and lemon juices, mustard, mint, garlic and salt; pour over greens and toss.

3. In shallow dish, stir together oil, curry paste, lemon juice, ginger and salt. Add shrimp and, using hands, toss to coat shrimp evenly. Place shrimp on greased grill over high heat and grill, turning once, for 4 minutes or until pink and firm. Add to greens.

Makes 3 servings.

—

Skewer Option: If the shrimp you purchase is small enough to fall through your grill, simply skewer them onto a bamboo or metal skewer and grill.

Skillet Option: If you don't have a grill, place the shrimp in a non-stick skillet over medium-high heat and cook for about 4 minutes or until pink and firm.

Meatless

Indian Vegetable Curry

So many wonderful vegetarian dishes come from India. This one has a smooth mild curry flavour, but you can spike up the heat by using a hot curry paste or powder. Serve this with basmati rice.

1 tbsp	canola oil
2	onions, cut in wedges
3	cloves garlic, minced
1 tbsp	chopped fresh ginger
1 tbsp	mild curry paste or powder
1 tsp	cumin seeds, crushed
3 cups	vegetable stock (low fat, low sodium)
2	red bell peppers, chopped
2 cups	broccoli florets
8 oz	green beans, cut into 1-inch pieces
1	zucchini, chopped
1	can (540 ml) chickpeas, drained and rinsed
¼ cup	chopped fresh coriander

—

1. In large saucepan, heat oil over medium heat. Cook onions, garlic, ginger, curry paste and cumin seeds for 5 minutes or until softened. Add stock and bring to boil. Add peppers, broccoli, beans, zucchini and chickpeas. Cover and simmer for about 15 minutes or until vegetables are tender-crisp. Sprinkle with coriander.

Makes 4 servings.

—

Lentil and Rice Filled Peppers   GREEN-LIGHT

Stuffed peppers have been around for a long time, and they still make a great meal. You can use any colour of bell pepper that you like.

1¼ cups	vegetable or chicken stock (low fat, low sodium)
¾ cup	brown rice
¼ tsp	salt
¼ tsp	dried thyme
1	small carrot, shredded
Half	zucchini, shredded
2 tbsp	chopped fresh parsley
¾ cup	low-fat pasta sauce
1	egg
2 tbsp	grated Parmesan cheese
1	can (540 ml) lentils, drained and rinsed
4	large red, green or yellow bell peppers
½ cup	water

—

1. In pot, bring stock, rice, salt and thyme to boil. Reduce heat to low, cover and cook for 25 minutes or until liquid is absorbed. Remove from heat and sprinkle carrot and zucchini on top of rice; cover and let steam for 5 minutes or until carrot is tender-crisp. Scrape rice into large bowl, add parsley and fluff with fork.

2. In small bowl, whisk together ½ cup of the pasta sauce, egg and cheese. Pour over rice and toss to combine. Add lentils and toss with mixture; set aside.

3. Cut top off each pepper. Remove seeds and ribs. Trim bottom of peppers to make them flat. Set peppers into 8-inch square baking dish. Pack each pepper with lentil and rice mixture. Spread remaining pasta sauce on top of peppers. Pour water into dish and cover with aluminum foil. Bake in 375°F oven for 40 minutes. Remove foil and return to oven and bake for 20 minutes or until bubbly and peppers are tender.

Makes 4 servings.

—

Bean Options: Try using beans, like black or pinto, instead of the lentils. Remember to drain and rinse them before using.

Ratatouille

Ratatouille is a hearty and pleasing vegetable stew. If there are any leftovers, add more vegetable stock to make a great chunky soup.

1 tbsp	olive oil
1	onion, chopped
4	cloves garlic, minced
Half	fennel bulb, diced
½ tsp	each dried basil and oregano
1	can (796 ml) diced tomatoes
2 cups	vegetable stock (low fat, low sodium)
2 cups	diced eggplant
2	zucchini, chopped
1	red bell pepper, chopped
2	cans (540 ml each) mixed beans, drained and rinsed
1 cup	diced firm tofu
¼ cup	chopped fresh Italian parsley
¼ tsp	each salt and pepper

—

1. In large soup pot, heat oil over medium-high heat. Cook onion, garlic, fennel, basil and oregano for 5 minutes or until they start to brown. Add tomatoes and stock and bring to boil.

2. Add eggplant, zucchini, red pepper, beans and tofu; return to boil. Reduce heat to simmer and cook for about 30 minutes or until slightly thickened and eggplant is very tender. Add parsley, salt and pepper.

Makes 4 servings.

—

Sweet-and-Sour Tofu

Sweet-and-sour sauce can often be sickly sweet without enough sour or heat to it. This version, however, is well-balanced and offers a great blanket of flavour for tofu, which can be rather bland. This dish is also good with chicken or pork.

1	pkg (350 g) extra-firm tofu
1 tbsp	canola oil
¼ cup	unsweetened pineapple juice
¼ cup	red wine vinegar
¼ cup	minced red bell pepper
3 tbsp	sugar substitute
1 tbsp	soy sauce
1	clove garlic, minced
2 tsp	minced fresh ginger
2 tsp	cornstarch

1. Cut tofu in half horizontally. Cut each half into 1/2-inch cubes. In non-stick skillet, heat oil over medium-high heat. Cook tofu for 10 minutes or until browned. Drain tofu on paper towel–lined plate; set aside.

2. In saucepan, whisk together juice, vinegar, red pepper, sugar substitute, soy sauce, garlic, ginger and cornstarch. Cook over medium heat, whisking occasionally, for about 5 minutes or until thickened and bubbly. Add tofu to sauce and toss to coat.

Makes 4 servings.

—

Helpful Hint: If extra-firm tofu is unavailable, simply drain firm tofu and place on a paper towel–lined plate. Top with another plate and a heavy can as a weight. Place in refrigerator for 4 hours, checking intermittently to drain any liquid. Then proceed with recipe.

Fettuccine Primavera GREEN-LIGHT

Primavera *means "springtime" in Italian, and you can use your favourite spring vegetables, such as asparagus or fiddleheads, in this pasta. Fortunately, you can get peppers, tomatoes and peas year-round, so you can make this dish any time.*

¼ cup	extra-virgin olive oil
2 cups	cubed firm tofu
3	cloves garlic, minced
¼ tsp	red pepper flakes
½ cup	vegetable cocktail juice
2 cups	chopped fresh asparagus or peas
1	red bell pepper, thinly sliced
1	carrot, julienned
1	yellow zucchini, thinly sliced
6 oz	whole wheat fettuccine or linguine pasta
2	plum tomatoes, chopped
¼ cup	chopped fresh Italian parsley
2 tbsp	grated Parmesan cheese

—

1. In non-stick skillet, heat 2 tbsp of the oil over medium-high heat. Brown tofu on all sides for about 2 minutes; remove to plate. Reserve oil.

2. In large shallow saucepan, heat remaining oil and reserved oil over medium heat. Cook garlic and red pepper flakes for 1 minute. Add vegetable cocktail juice; bring to boil. Reduce heat and simmer for 1 minute. Add asparagus, red pepper, carrot and zucchini; cook, stirring, for 10 minutes or until vegetables are tender-crisp.

3. Meanwhile, in large pot of boiling salted water, cook fettuccine for 8 minutes or until al dente. Drain and return to pot. Add vegetables, tofu and toss to coat. Stir in tomatoes, parsley and cheese.

Makes 4 servings.

—

Asian Greens and Tofu Stir-fry GREEN-LIGHT

The wide variety of Asian greens available in grocery stores these days provides excellent new options for old stir-fries. Shanghai bok choy is all green while the stalks of baby bok choy are white. Serve this with egg or rice noodles.

4	green onions
2 tsp	canola oil
4	baby bok choy, chopped coarsely
2	Shanghai bok choy, chopped coarsely
2	carrots, shredded
1	red bell pepper, thinly sliced
¼ cup	vegetable stock or water
2 tbsp	soy sauce
½ tsp	toasted sesame oil
1	pkg (500 g) firm tofu, drained and cubed
1	clove garlic, minced
1 tbsp	minced fresh ginger
1 tbsp	rice vinegar
1 tbsp	sesame seeds, toasted

—

1. Chop green onions, separating the white part from the green. Set green parts aside.

2. In non-stick skillet or wok, heat oil over medium-high heat and cook white parts of green onions for 30 seconds. Add baby and Shanghai bok choy, carrots and pepper. Stir-fry for 5 minutes. Add stock, soy sauce and sesame oil; bring to boil. Add tofu, garlic and ginger. Reduce heat to medium; cover and cook for 3 minutes or until vegetables are tender-crisp.

3. Drizzle vegetables with vinegar and sprinkle with sesame seeds and reserved green onions.

Makes 4 servings.

—

Bulgur and Chickpea Chili

Bulgur takes the place of meat in this satisfying vegetarian chili. You can find bulgur, which is also known as cracked wheat, in bulk and health food stores.

1 tbsp	canola oil
1	onion, chopped
4	cloves garlic, minced
2	celery stalks, chopped
1	carrot, chopped
1 tbsp	chili powder
1 tbsp	dried oregano
1 tsp	ground cumin
2	cans (796 ml each) diced tomatoes
1 cup	vegetable stock (low fat, low sodium)
2	cans (540 ml each) chickpeas, drained and rinsed
¾ cup	bulgur
1	red bell pepper, chopped
¼ tsp	each salt and pepper

—

1. In large pot, heat oil over medium heat. Cook onion, garlic, celery, carrot, chili powder, oregano and cumin for about 5 minutes or until softened. Add tomatoes and vegetable stock; bring to boil. Add chickpeas and bulgur; reduce heat and simmer for about 20 minutes or until bulgur is tender. Add red pepper, salt and pepper and cook for another 10 minutes or until thickened.

Makes 4 to 6 servings.

—

Rice Option: You can substitute brown, basmati or long-grain rice for the bulgur, but increase cooking time to 30 minutes.

Easy Bake Lasagna

Though cooking the G.I. way usually means starting from scratch, there are some handy convenience products that are low G.I., such as pasta sauce! This lasagna is great for a crowd. All you need to go with it is a tossed salad.

12	whole wheat lasagna noodles
2 tsp	canola oil
1	onion, chopped
1	red bell pepper, chopped
8 oz	mushrooms, sliced
¼ tsp	each salt and pepper
1	bag (300 g) baby spinach
1½ cups	diced firm tofu
1 cup	1% cottage cheese
⅓ cup	liquid egg
1	jar (700 mL) low-fat pasta sauce
1½ cups	shredded part-skim mozzarella cheese
2 tbsp	grated Parmesan cheese

—

1. In large pot of boiling salted water, cook lasagna noodles for about 10 minutes or until al dente. Drain and rinse under cold water. Lay noodles flat on damp tea towels; set aside.

2. Meanwhile, in large non-stick skillet, heat oil over medium-high heat. Cook onion, red pepper, mushrooms, salt and pepper for about 8 minutes or until golden brown and liquid is evaporated. Add spinach and cook, stirring, for 2 minutes or until wilted. Stir in tofu. In small bowl, stir together cottage cheese and liquid egg; set aside.

3. Ladle ½ cup of the pasta sauce in bottom of 9- x 13-inch glass baking dish. Lay 3 noodles on top of sauce. Spread one third of the spinach mixture over top and one third of the cottage cheese mixture. Spread with another ½ cup of the pasta sauce. Sprinkle with ⅓ cup of the mozzarella. Repeat layers, ending with noodles on top. Spread with remaining sauce and sprinkle with remaining mozzarella and Parmesan cheeses. Cover with aluminum foil and bake in 350°F oven for 45 minutes. Uncover and bake for 15 minutes or until bubbly and knife inserted in centre is hot to the touch. Let cool 10 minutes before cutting and serving.

Makes 8 servings.

—

Storage: You can assemble the lasagna and refrigerate it for up to 1 day before baking. You can freeze the baked lasagna whole or in portions and reheat in the microwave.

Fish and Seafood

Cornmeal-Crusted Pickerel GREEN-LIGHT

Cornmeal provides a crunchy, almost nutty texture to fish. Try any of your favourite fillets, such as cod or tilapia, in this dish——pickerel is one of my favourites. Serve with broccoli spears and Tangy Red and Green Coleslaw (see recipe page 146).

1 cup	cornmeal
2 tbsp	chopped fresh dill or 2 tsp dried dillweed
1 tbsp	grated Parmesan cheese
1/4 tsp	each salt and pepper
Pinch	cayenne
4	fish fillets (pickerel, cod or tilapia), each 4 oz
1	egg, lightly beaten
2 tbsp	canola oil

—

1. In large shallow dish or pie plate, combine cornmeal, dill, Parmesan, salt, pepper and cayenne; set aside.

2. Pat fish fillets dry using paper towels. Brush each fillet with egg and then dip into cornmeal mixture, turning to coat both sides well.

3. In large non-stick skillet, heat oil over medium-high heat. Cook fish fillets for 3 minutes. Using spatula, carefully turn fillets and cook for another 3 minutes or until fish flakes easily with fork.

Makes 4 servings.

—

Almond Haddock Fillets   GREEN-LIGHT

*Almonds provide calcium to this fish dish. Serve with Lemon Dill
Lentil Salad (see recipe page 154), green beans and rice.*

½ cup	almonds
¼ cup	fresh whole wheat bread crumbs
2 tbsp	chopped fresh tarragon or 1 tsp dried
1 tsp	grated lemon rind
¼ tsp	each salt and pepper
1 tbsp	canola oil
4	haddock fillets, each 4 oz
	Lemon wedges

—

1. Place almonds in food processor; pulse until almonds resemble coarse bread crumbs. Remove to large pie plate or shallow dish. Add bread crumbs, tarragon, lemon rind, salt and pepper and combine.

2. Pat fillets dry using paper towels. Brush some of the oil over fish. Dredge in nut mixture to coat both sides.

3. In non-stick skillet, heat remaining oil over medium-high heat. Brown fish on both sides. Place fillets on parchment paper– or aluminum foil–lined baking sheet and roast in 425°F oven for about 10 minutes or until fish just flakes with fork. Serve with lemon wedges.

Makes 4 servings.

—

Helpful Hint: If you can't find haddock, look for other great whitefish like halibut, cod, tilapia or whiting. You can also try this mixture on salmon or catfish fillets.

Tuna Patty Melts

Make these for lunch at home, or omit the cheese and pack them up for the office. Enjoy with the Creamy Cucumber or Lemon Dill Lentil salads (see recipes on pages 143 and 154).

2	cans (120 g each) chunk white tuna, drained
1	dill pickle, finely chopped
¼ cup	light mayonnaise
¼ tsp	grated lemon rind
2 tsp	lemon juice
2 tbsp	finely chopped celery
2 tbsp	diced red bell pepper
¼ tsp	each salt and pepper
2	whole wheat English muffins
4	slices light-style Cheddar cheese

—

1. In bowl, combine tuna, pickle, mayonnaise, lemon rind and juice, celery, red pepper, salt and pepper; set aside.

2. Toast English muffins in toaster or under broiler. Divide tuna mixture among muffins. Top with cheese. Place under broiler for 30 seconds or until melted.

Makes 4 servings.

—

Bread Option: You can serve this tuna mixture on 4 slices of stone-ground whole wheat bread if you like.

Tomato-Topped Shrimp

Serve this shrimp with rice to sop up all the tomato juices. Brighten up your plate with some asparagus and Mediterranean Bean Salad (see recipe page 152).

2 tsp	extra-virgin olive oil
1	onion, finely chopped
4	cloves garlic, minced
¼ cup	chopped fresh basil or Italian parsley
½ tsp	dried oregano
Pinch	red pepper flakes
¼ cup	dry white wine or chicken stock
2	tomatoes, diced
½ cup	coarsely chopped cooked chickpeas
¼ tsp	each salt and pepper
8 oz	medium raw shrimp, peeled and deveined, or bay scallops

—

1. In non-stick skillet, heat oil over medium-high heat. Cook onion, garlic, 3 tbsp of the basil, oregano and red pepper flakes for 5 minutes or until they start to become golden. Add wine and cook for 1 minute.

2. Add tomatoes, chickpeas, salt and pepper. Cook for about 8 minutes or until mixture starts to thicken. Add shrimp and cook for 4 minutes or until pink and firm. Sprinkle with remaining basil.

Makes 2 servings.

—

Helpful Hint: The wine in this recipe gives a slightly tangy flavour to the sauce. If you use chicken stock, add ½ tsp wine vinegar or cider vinegar to the finished sauce before adding the shrimp.

Salmon Steaks
with Light Dill Tartar Sauce GREEN-LIGHT

The marinade and sauce also go well with other fish, such as halibut, bluefish or tilapia. Round out the meal with rice and mixed vegetables.

1 tsp	canola oil
1	clove garlic, minced
2 tsp	grated lemon rind
2 tbsp	lemon juice
1 tsp	Dijon mustard
½ tsp	each salt and pepper
4	salmon steaks, each 4 oz

Light Dill Tartar Sauce:

¼ cup	non-fat plain yogurt
¼ cup	light mayonnaise
2 tbsp	chopped fresh dill or 2 tsp dried dillweed
1 tbsp	capers, chopped
1	dill pickle, finely chopped
1	green onion, finely chopped

—

1. In bowl, whisk together oil, garlic, lemon rind and juice, mustard, salt and pepper. Coat salmon steaks with mixture; let stand for 15 minutes.

2. Light Dill Tartar Sauce: In another bowl, whisk together yogurt, mayonnaise, dill, capers, pickle and green onion. Cover and refrigerate until ready to use.

3. Place salmon on greased grill over medium-high heat and grill for 10 minutes, turning once, or until fish just flakes with fork. Serve with Light Dill Tartar Sauce.

Makes 4 servings.

—

Sesame Scallop and Black Bean Toss

GREEN-LIGHT

Scallops are rich in protein and zinc, but if they are unavailable, you can use jumbo shrimp that have been peeled and deveined.

2 tbsp	sesame seeds
8 oz	sea scallops
2 tsp	canola oil
½ cup	thinly sliced red onion
1	clove garlic, minced
2 cups	broccoli florets
1	orange or red bell pepper, sliced
1 cup	cooked black beans
2 tbsp	hoisin sauce
¼ cup	orange juice
½ tsp	sesame oil
Pinch	each salt and pepper
¼ cup	chopped fresh coriander (optional)

—

1. Place sesame seeds on plate. Coat sides of each scallop with seeds; set aside.

2. In large non-stick skillet, heat oil over medium-high heat. Brown scallops on all sides and remove to plate; cover to keep warm. Leave remaining sesame seeds in skillet.

3. In same skillet, reduce heat to medium and cook onion and garlic for 3 minutes. Add broccoli, orange pepper, beans, hoisin sauce, orange juice, sesame oil, salt and pepper; cook for about 8 minutes or until broccoli is tender-crisp. Return scallops to skillet and heat through. Sprinkle with coriander (if using).

Makes 2 servings.

—

Hoisin Orange
Halibut Steak Packets

The flavours of hoisin sauce and orange go well together and provide a delicious sauce for delicate halibut.

4	baby bok choy, coarsely chopped
8 oz	shiitake mushrooms, sliced
1	red bell pepper, sliced
2	cloves garlic, slivered
2 tsp	canola oil
¼ tsp	each salt and pepper
2	halibut steaks, each 4 oz
¼ cup	hoisin sauce
1 tsp	grated orange rind
¼ cup	orange juice
1 tbsp	chopped fresh Italian parsley

—

1. In bowl, combine bok choy, mushrooms, red pepper, garlic, oil, salt and pepper. Divide vegetables between 2 pieces of aluminum foil. Top each portion with a halibut steak.

2. In small bowl, combine hoisin sauce, orange rind and juice and parsley. Drizzle over each halibut steak. Top with another piece of aluminum foil and seal to form packets. Place on greased grill over medium-high heat, or in 425°F oven, for about 20 minutes or until fish flakes easily with fork, vegetables are tender, and foil packages puff slightly.

Makes 2 servings.

—

Helpful Hint: You can substitute tilapia, sole or haddock for the halibut.

Grilled Pesto Salmon
with Asparagus

GREEN-LIGHT

A little bit of store-bought pesto can add a lot of flavour to your food. Here it is combined with mayonnaise to form a decadent but light crust for salmon. I've received rave reviews for this recipe in my cooking classes.

¼ cup	light mayonnaise
2 tbsp	chopped fresh Italian parsley
1 tbsp	pesto
Pinch	each salt and pepper
4	boneless salmon fillets, skin on, each 4 oz

Grilled Asparagus:

1 lb	asparagus spears
2 tsp	extra-virgin olive oil
¼ tsp	pepper
2 tbsp	lemon juice
¼ tsp	salt

—

1. In small bowl, whisk together mayonnaise, parsley, pesto, salt and pepper. Spread evenly over top of salmon.

2. Grilled Asparagus: Snap tough ends of asparagus off and discard. Toss spears with oil and pepper.

3. Place fillets and asparagus on greased grill over medium-high heat. Close lid and grill for about 10 minutes or until fish is firm to the touch and asparagus is tender-crisp. Drizzle asparagus with lemon juice and sprinkle with salt.

Makes 4 servings.

—

Fish Options: This pesto mixture is delicious on halibut, marlin, tuna or trout.

Helpful Hint: Leaving the skin on the fillets helps the fish stay moist and keeps it from falling apart.

Garlic Shrimp Pasta

GREEN-LIGHT

Garlic is heart healthy because it helps to reduce cholesterol and is a great decongestant, too. Don't be afraid of the amount of garlic in this dish—the flavour softens as it cooks.

1 tbsp	extra-virgin olive oil
6	cloves garlic, minced
¼ tsp	red pepper flakes
½ cup	dry white wine or chicken stock
1 lb	large raw shrimp, peeled and deveined
½ cup	chopped fresh Italian parsley
1 tbsp	non-hydrogenated soft margarine
6 oz	whole wheat linguine or fettuccine

—

1. In large non-stick skillet, heat oil over medium heat and cook garlic and red pepper flakes for 1 minute or until garlic starts to turn golden. Add wine and bring to boil. Add shrimp and cook for 5 minutes or until shrimp are pink and firm. Add parsley and margarine and cook until melted.

2. Meanwhile, in large pot of boiling salted water, cook pasta for 8 minutes or until al dente. Drain and add to shrimp mixture. Toss to coat with sauce.

Makes 4 servings.

—

Leek-Stuffed Sole

GREEN-LIGHT

Tender leek stuffing gives this fish a burst of flavour. Lemon, olives and tomato add a touch of the Mediterranean.

1 tbsp	extra-virgin olive oil
3	leeks, white and light green parts only, chopped
3	cloves garlic, minced
1 tbsp	grated lemon rind
1 tbsp	chopped fresh dill or 1 tsp dried dillweed
4	sole fillets, each 4 oz
¼ tsp	each salt and pepper
1	tomato, diced
3 tbsp	chopped black olives
2 tbsp	lemon juice

—

1. In non-stick skillet, heat oil over medium heat. Cook leeks and garlic for about 15 minutes, stirring occasionally, or until softened and golden. Stir in lemon rind, dill and half each of the salt and pepper. Let cool slightly.

2. Place ¼ cup of the leek mixture on bottom of small casserole dish. Place some of the remaining leek mixture in centre of each sole fillet; gently fold fillet over filling. Lay stuffed sole in dish. Sprinkle each fillet with remaining salt and pepper.

3. In small bowl, combine tomato, olives and lemon juice. Sprinkle over sole. Bake in 425°F oven for about 15 minutes or until fish just flakes with fork.

Makes 4 servings.

—

Helpful Hint: To clean leeks, simply cut dark green part off and remove any outer layers. Trim root end. Cut leek in half lengthwise and rinse under water to remove any dirt. Pat dry and chop.

Ginger Salmon in Parchment   GREEN-LIGHT

Cooking in parchment—en papillote—is an easy, healthful way to prepare fish and keeps in all its moisture and flavour. I find that guests enjoy opening their own packages at the table for a "surprise" dinner.

4 cups	shredded napa cabbage
1	red bell pepper, thinly sliced
1 cup	snow peas, halved
4	salmon fillets, skin removed, each 4 oz
¼ cup	soy sauce
2	green onions, chopped
1 tbsp	minced fresh ginger
1	clove garlic, minced
1 tsp	sesame oil
¼ tsp	pepper

—

1. Cut four large pieces of parchment paper and fold each in half. Then unfold them and set aside.

2. Combine cabbage, red pepper and snow peas. Divide vegetables evenly on one side of the fold of each piece of parchment paper. Place salmon fillets on top of vegetables.

3. In small bowl, whisk together soy sauce, green onions, ginger, garlic, sesame oil and pepper. Drizzle over fish and vegetables. Fold empty half of parchment over and fold edges to seal. Place packages on large baking sheet and bake in 400°F oven for about 20 minutes or until fish flakes easily with fork.

Makes 4 servings.

—

Helpful Hint: If you don't have parchment, you can still make these delicious packages with aluminum foil.

Fish Options: Try this recipe with any of your favourite fish, such as halibut, tilapia or snapper.

Poultry

Coriander Ginger Turkey Burgers

GREEN-LIGHT

You can serve these on whole wheat bun halves, but they are just as tasty on their own. If ground turkey is unavailable, you can use ground chicken.

1	egg, lightly beaten
2 tbsp	soy sauce
2	green onions, chopped
2	cloves garlic, minced
1 tbsp	minced fresh ginger
⅓ cup	chopped fresh coriander
⅓ cup	crushed whole wheat crackers or dry bread crumbs
¼ tsp	pepper
1 lb	lean ground turkey

—

1. In large bowl, whisk together egg and soy sauce. Stir in onions, garlic, ginger, coriander, crushed crackers and pepper. Add turkey and, using hands, mix into egg mixture until evenly distributed. Shape into 4 patties about ½-inch thick.

2. Place patties in large non-stick skillet over medium-high heat; cover and cook, turning once, for about 15 minutes, or until no longer pink inside.

Makes 4 servings.

—

Turkey and Snow Pea Stir-fry   GREEN-LIGHT

Now that turkey has become more readily available in supermarkets throughout the year, it's not just for the holidays any more. You can use it instead of chicken in any recipe. In this stir-fry, the turkey takes on a great lemony flavour.

1 lb	boneless skinless turkey breasts or stir-fry strips
½ tsp	each dried sage and thyme leaves
½ tsp	salt
¼ tsp	pepper
2 tsp	canola oil
3	green onions, chopped
2	cloves garlic, minced
1	red bell pepper, chopped
2 cups	snow peas, halved
½ cup	chicken stock
½ tsp	grated lemon rind
1 tbsp	lemon juice

—

1. Cut turkey into bite-size pieces. Sprinkle with half each of the sage, thyme, salt and pepper.

2. In large non-stick skillet, heat oil over medium-high heat; cook turkey for 8 minutes or until no longer pink inside. Remove to plate and keep warm.

3. Return skillet to heat and cook onions, garlic and red pepper with remaining sage, thyme, salt and pepper for 5 minutes or until softened. Add snow peas, stock and lemon rind. Bring to boil, cover and cook for 1 minute or until snow peas are tender-crisp. Return turkey to pan and heat through. Drizzle with lemon juice.

Makes 4 servings.

—

Grilled Rosemary
Chicken Thighs

GREEN-LIGHT

Chicken thighs are cheaper than breasts but are more flavourful and very tender. If it isn't barbecue season, bake them in a 400°F oven for about twenty minutes.

2 tbsp	extra-virgin olive oil
2	cloves garlic, minced
2 tsp	grated lemon rind
2 tbsp	lemon juice
2 tbsp	dry white wine
2 tbsp	chopped fresh rosemary or
	2 tsp dried rosemary, crushed
¼ tsp	salt
8	boneless skinless chicken thighs

—

1. In bowl, whisk together oil, garlic, lemon rind and juice, wine, rosemary and salt. Add chicken thighs and toss to coat. Cover and refrigerate for 15 to 30 minutes.

2. Place thighs on greased grill over medium-high heat. Close lid and grill, turning once, for about 20 minutes, or until juices run clear when pierced with knife.

Makes 4 servings.

—

Helpful Hint: You can use 1 tbsp white wine vinegar or cider vinegar instead of the wine.

Lemon Yogurt Chicken   GREEN-LIGHT

This has been adapted from a recipe that Lenna F. sent to us via e-mail. The yogurt marinade keeps the chicken breasts juicy and flavourful. Serve them with Lentil and Rice Filled Peppers (see recipe page 170).

1 cup	non-fat plain yogurt
1 tsp	grated lemon rind
1 tbsp	lemon juice
1	clove garlic, minced
Pinch	each salt and pepper
4	boneless skinless chicken breasts

—

1. In large shallow dish, whisk together yogurt, lemon rind and juice, garlic, salt and pepper. Add chicken breasts and turn to coat with yogurt mixture. Cover and refrigerate for at least 1 hour or overnight.

2. Remove excess yogurt from chicken and discard. Place chicken breasts on greased grill over medium-high heat. Close lid and grill, turning once, for about 12 minutes or until no longer pink inside.

Makes 4 servings.

—

Hunter-Style Chicken

*Ubiquitously known as Chicken Cacciatore, cacciatore meaning
"hunter" in Italian, this dish is a favourite among adults and kids
alike. You can use all drumsticks or all thighs if you like.*

1 lb	skinless chicken drumsticks
1 lb	skinless chicken thighs
¼ tsp	each salt and pepper
2 tbsp	extra-virgin olive oil
1	onion, chopped
4	cloves garlic, minced
1 lb	mushrooms, quartered
1	each red and green bell peppers, chopped
1 tbsp	dried oregano
1 tsp	dried basil
¼ cup	dry white wine or chicken stock
1	can (796 ml) diced tomatoes

—

1. Sprinkle salt and pepper all over chicken pieces. In large shallow pot, heat half of the oil over medium-high heat and brown chicken on both sides. Remove to plate.

2. In same pot, heat remaining oil over medium-high heat and cook onion, garlic, mushrooms, peppers, oregano and basil for about 15 minutes or until vegetables are beginning to brown. Pour in wine and stir vegetables to deglaze pan. Add tomatoes and bring to boil. Return chicken to pot. Reduce heat; simmer for 45 minutes or until chicken is starting to fall off the bone.

Makes 6 servings.

—

Thai Chicken Curry

GREEN-LIGHT

You can use any colour—green, red or yellow—of Thai curry paste in this hot and spicy dish. If you want it extra hot, increase the curry paste to 1 tablespoon.

1 tbsp	canola oil
2 tsp	red Thai curry paste
1 lb	boneless skinless chicken breasts, cut in chunks
1	onion, sliced
1	each red and green bell peppers, thinly sliced
½ cup	chicken stock or water
½ cup	light coconut milk or light sour cream
2 tbsp	fish or soy sauce
¼ cup	chopped fresh basil or coriander

—

1. In large skillet or wok, heat oil over medium-high heat. Add curry paste and cook for 30 seconds. Add chicken and stir-fry for 5 minutes. Add onion and peppers; cook, stirring, for about 10 minutes or until vegetables begin to brown. Add stock, coconut milk and fish sauce; simmer for 10 minutes or until chicken is no longer pink inside. Stir in basil.

Makes 4 servings.

—

Vegetarian Option: You can substitute 2 pkgs (350 g each) extra-firm tofu, cubed, for the chicken, and soy sauce for the fish sauce.

Beef Option: You can substitute 1 lb top sirloin grilling steak, thinly sliced, for the chicken, and beef stock for the chicken stock.

Ginger Chicken

Ginger adds a wonderful fresh flavour to this chicken dish. The corian-der, cumin and turmeric give it a beautiful sunny yellow colour.

2 tbsp	canola oil
2 tbsp	grated fresh ginger
1 tsp	ground coriander
½ tsp	ground cumin
½ tsp	turmeric
¾ tsp	salt
¼ tsp	pepper
1 ½ lb	skinless chicken pieces
4 cups	cauliflower florets
2	carrots, cut in chunks
1	red onion, cut in wedges

—

1. In small bowl, combine 1 tbsp of the oil, the ginger, coriander, cumin, turmeric, ¼ tsp of the salt, and a pinch of the pepper. Rub mixture all over chicken.

2. Toss cauliflower, carrots and onion with remaining oil, salt and pepper. Place chicken and vegetables on parchment paper–lined baking sheet or roasting pan. Roast in 425°F oven for about 35 minutes or until juices run clear when chicken is pierced and vegetables are tender-crisp and golden.

Makes 4 servings.

—

Orange and Chicken Stew   GREEN-LIGHT

This dish is based on chicken à l'Orange, which was a popular dish for entertaining in the seventies. It is easy to prepare and has a rich orangey flavour. Serve with rice and a tossed salad.

2 tsp	canola oil
1 lb	boneless skinless chicken breasts, cut into bite-size pieces
2	onions, chopped
2	cloves garlic, minced
8 oz	mushrooms, sliced
1 tbsp	chopped fresh rosemary or 1 tsp dried
1 tbsp	chopped fresh thyme leaves or 1 tsp dried
¼ tsp	each salt and pepper
2 tsp	grated orange rind
2	oranges, peeled and chopped
1 cup	chicken stock (low fat, low sodium)
1	bay leaf
1	can (540 ml) Romano beans, drained and rinsed
1	green bell pepper, chopped
1 tbsp	cider vinegar
⅓ cup	chopped fresh Italian parsley
2 tsp	cornstarch
1 tbsp	water

—

1. In large deep non-stick skillet, heat oil over medium-high heat. Brown chicken and remove to plate. In same skillet, add onions, garlic, mushrooms, rosemary, thyme, salt and pepper and cook for 8 minutes or until liquid is evaporated. Return chicken to skillet with orange rind, oranges, stock and bay leaf. Bring to boil. Cover and simmer for about 30 minutes or until chicken is no longer pink inside.

2. Add beans, green pepper, vinegar and parsley; cook for 10 minutes or until heated through. In small bowl, whisk together cornstarch and water. Stir into stew and cook until slightly thickened. Remove bay leaf.

Makes 4 servings.

—

Yellow-Light Pork Option: You can substitute boneless pork loin for the chicken.

Chicken Enchiladas

I love having themed dinners, and this recipe is perfect for a Mexican fiesta. Serve these enchiladas with low-fat refried beans and rice for a fun party meal.

2 tbsp	canola oil
2 tsp	chili powder
1 tsp	ground cumin
1 tsp	dried oregano
¼ tsp	each salt and pepper
4	boneless skinless chicken breasts, cut into bite-size pieces
2	onions, sliced
1	each red and green bell peppers, thinly sliced
1	jalapeno pepper, seeded and minced
1 cup	drained diced tomatoes
½ cup	shredded light-style Cheddar or Monterey Jack cheese
8	large whole wheat tortillas

Toppings:

½ cup	shredded light-style Cheddar or Monterey Jack cheese
½ cup	light sour cream

—

1. In bowl, combine 1 tbsp of the canola oil, the chili powder, cumin, oregano, salt and pepper. Add chicken and coat with mixture. In non-stick skillet, heat remaining oil over medium-high heat; cook chicken for about 10 minutes or until no longer pink inside. Remove to plate.

2. Reduce heat to medium and cook onions, red and green peppers and jalapeno in same skillet for about 10 minutes or until tender; set aside.

3. Add chicken, tomatoes and cheese to pepper mixture; stir to combine. Divide filling among tortillas and roll up. Place in shallow 9- x 13-inch greased baking dish. Cover with aluminum foil and bake in 400°F oven for about 15 minutes or until filling is hot. Remove foil and bake for another 5 minutes or until tortillas are crisp. Sprinkle with cheese and dollop with sour cream before serving.

Makes 4 servings.

—

Beef Option: You can substitute 1 lb of top sirloin grilling steak, thinly sliced, for the chicken.

Shrimp Option: You can substitute 1 lb large raw shrimp, peeled and deveined, for the chicken.

Meat

Beef and Eggplant Chili

The addition of eggplant gives this chili a delicious twist. Sprinkle with light-style Monterey Jack cheese for extra zip.

12 oz	extra-lean ground beef
1 tbsp	canola oil
2	onions, chopped
4	cloves garlic, minced
2 tbsp	chili powder
1 tbsp	dried oregano
1 tsp	ground cumin
2	green bell peppers, chopped
2 cups	diced eggplant
1	can (796 ml) diced tomatoes
½ cup	tomato paste
1	can (540 ml) red kidney beans, drained and rinsed

—

1. In large saucepan over medium-high heat, brown beef and remove to plate. In same saucepan, heat oil over medium heat and add onions, garlic, chili powder, oregano and cumin, stirring for about 5 minutes or until softened. Add peppers and eggplant; cook for 10 minutes or until lightly golden. Add tomatoes, tomato paste and browned beef; bring to boil. Reduce heat and add beans. Simmer for about 1 hour or until eggplant is very tender.

Makes 4 servings.

Horseradish Burgers   GREEN-LIGHT

The combination of beef and horseradish makes these burgers a hit with meat lovers. For a spicier horseradish flavour, simply smother the top with some more horseradish. Serve with a side of Tabbouleh Salad (see recipe page 157).

1	small onion, grated
1	clove garlic, minced
2 tbsp	horseradish
2 tbsp	steak sauce
1 tbsp	Dijon mustard
1 tbsp	Worcestershire sauce
2 tsp	dried oregano
½ tsp	pepper
¼ tsp	salt
2 tbsp	wheat bran
2 tbsp	wheat germ
1 lb	extra-lean ground beef
2	whole wheat buns
4	leaves lettuce
1	tomato, sliced
¼ cup	alfalfa sprouts (optional)

—

1. In large bowl, stir together onion, garlic, horseradish, steak sauce, mustard, Worcestershire, oregano, pepper and salt. Add bran and wheat germ; stir to coat. Let stand for 5 minutes. Using hands, mix in beef until mixture is well combined.

2. Form meat mixture into 4 patties about ½-inch thick. Place on greased grill or in non-stick skillet and grill or cook, turning once, for about 12 minutes, or until no longer pink inside. Place patties on each half of buns. Top with lettuce, tomato slices and sprouts (if using).

Makes 4 servings.

—

Beef Fajitas

Here is a restaurant classic that is simple to make at home! Serve the fajitas sizzling from the skillet for great effect.

1 tsp	canola oil
8 oz	top sirloin grilling steak, thinly sliced
1 tbsp	Worcestershire sauce
Pinch	cayenne
1	red onion, sliced
2	cloves garlic, minced
1	each red and green bell peppers, sliced
2 tsp	chili powder
½ tsp	each ground cumin and dried thyme
¼ tsp	each salt and pepper
¼ cup	low-fat pasta sauce or low-fat salsa
4	small whole wheat tortillas
¼ cup	light sour cream

—

1. In large non-stick skillet, heat oil over medium-high heat. Cook steak, Worcestershire sauce and cayenne for 5 minutes or until browned. Remove to plate.

2. Return skillet to medium heat and cook onion, garlic, red and green peppers, chili powder, cumin, thyme, salt and pepper for 8 minutes or until tender-crisp. Add pasta sauce and cook for 5 minutes. Return beef to pan and cook until heated through.

3. Divide meat mixture among tortillas, dollop with some sour cream and roll up.

Makes 2 servings.

—

Chicken/Turkey Option: You can use boneless skinless chicken or turkey breast instead of the beef.

Serving Option: You can serve the meat mixture over rice instead of filling the tortillas.

Beefy Meatballs

You can use ground pork, veal, chicken or turkey instead of the beef in this recipe. Serve the meatballs on their own or with your favourite low-fat pasta sauce and whole wheat spaghetti.

1	egg
½ cup	crushed whole-wheat crackers
⅓ cup	chopped fresh Italian parsley
2 tbsp	grated Parmesan cheese
2 tbsp	wheat germ or wheat bran
2	cloves garlic, minced
½ tsp	salt
¼ tsp	red pepper flakes
1 ½ lb	extra-lean ground beef

—

1. In large bowl, whisk egg with fork. Add crackers, parsley, cheese, wheat germ, garlic, salt and red pepper flakes; stir to combine. Add meat and combine well, using hands to distribute ingredients evenly.

2. Roll meat mixture into 1-inch balls and place on aluminum foil–lined baking sheet. Bake in 400°F oven for 20 minutes or until no longer pink inside.

Makes 6 servings or about 24 meatballs.

—

Mini Meatball Option: Use a teaspoon measure to make tiny meatballs for your family.

Storage: Let meatballs cool completely. Place in airtight container or resealable bag and freeze for up to 2 months.

Easy Meat Sauce

Half of this recipe served with 6 oz of whole wheat pasta makes a great dinner for four. You can also use this sauce in lasagna or even eat it on its own like chili.

12 oz	extra-lean ground beef
1 tbsp	canola oil
1	onion, chopped
2	cloves garlic, chopped
1 tbsp	dried oregano
1 tsp	salt
¼ tsp	red pepper flakes
2	cans (796 ml each) plum tomatoes, puréed
1	each red and green bell peppers, chopped
4	fresh basil leaves
4	sprigs fresh Italian parsley

—

1. In deep pot, cook beef over medium-high heat for about 8 minutes or until browned. Remove to plate; reduce heat to medium. In same pot, add oil, onion, garlic, oregano, salt and red pepper flakes; cook, stirring, for about 5 minutes or until softened.

2. Add tomatoes, peppers, basil and parsley and bring to boil. Return meat to sauce. Reduce heat and simmer for about 30 minutes or until thickened.

Makes about 5 ½ cups.

—

Storage: Let mixture cool completely and put in airtight containers. Freeze for up to 1 month.

Spicy Beef and Beans GREEN-LIGHT

This dish is mildly spicy and goes well with pasta and Tangy Red and Green Coleslaw (see recipe for 146).

1 lb	lean stewing beef
1 tbsp	canola oil
1	onion, chopped
1	carrot, chopped
2	cloves garlic, minced
8 oz	mushrooms, sliced
1 tsp	dried thyme leaves
½ tsp	red pepper flakes
2 cups	beef stock
¼ cup	tomato paste
1 tbsp	Worcestershire sauce
1	bay leaf
1	can (540 ml) white beans, drained and rinsed
1	red bell pepper, chopped
½ tsp	salt
¼ tsp	pepper
¼ cup	chopped fresh basil or parsley

—

1. In large shallow saucepan, heat some of the oil over medium-high heat and brown beef. Remove to plate; set aside.

2. Return saucepan to medium heat and add any remaining oil. Add onion, carrot, garlic, mushrooms, thyme and red pepper flakes; cook for about 8 minutes or until golden. Add beef stock, tomato paste, Worcestershire sauce, bay leaf and browned beef and juices. Bring to boil. Reduce heat, cover and simmer for 1 hour.

3. Uncover and add beans, red pepper, salt and pepper. Cover and return to simmer for 1 hour or until beef is very tender. Remove bay leaf. Stir in basil.

Makes 4 servings.

—

Yellow-Light Lamb Option: You can substitute lamb for the beef.

Lazy Cabbage Rolls

GREEN-LIGHT

Making traditional cabbage rolls can be a time-consuming process. If you aren't up to the task but want to enjoy the same great flavour, this is the dish for you. It has all the same ingredients but takes less than half the time to make.

2 tsp	canola oil
1	onion, finely chopped
2	garlic cloves, minced
¾ cup	basmati rice
1 ½ cups	beef or chicken stock (low fat, low sodium)
½ tsp	salt
¼ tsp	pepper
12 oz	extra-lean ground beef
½ tsp	fennel or caraway seeds, crushed
½ tsp	dried oregano
⅓ cup	liquid egg
¼ cup	chopped fresh Italian parsley
1	jar (700 ml) low-fat pasta sauce
6 cups	shredded cabbage
½ cup	water

—

1. In small pot, heat oil over medium heat. Cook onion and garlic for about 3 minutes or until softened. Add rice and stir to coat. Pour in beef stock and half each of the salt and pepper; bring to boil. Cover and reduce heat to low; cook for 15 minutes or until liquid is absorbed. Scrape rice into large bowl; fluff with fork. Set aside.

2. In non-stick skillet over medium-high heat, cook beef, fennel, oregano and remaining salt and pepper until browned and cooked through. Add to rice mixture; stir in liquid egg and parsley until combined.

3. Spread ½ cup of the pasta sauce over bottom of 9- x 13-inch baking dish. Sprinkle one third of the cabbage over bottom. Spread with half of the rice mixture. Spread with another ½ cup of the pasta sauce. Sprinkle with another third of the cabbage and remaining rice mixture. Finish with remaining cabbage, packing down gently. Spread remaining pasta sauce and water evenly over top. Cover with aluminum foil and bake in 350°F oven for about 1 hour or until cabbage is tender.

Makes 6 servings.

—

Poultry Options: You can substitute ground chicken or turkey for the beef.

Fennel Option: You can use a combination of ¼ tsp anise seeds, crushed, and ¼ tsp celery seeds, if you don't have fennel.

Veal Parmesan

Traditionally, this classic Italian dish is made with breaded, fried veal. I've lightened it up by omitting the bread crumbs and grilling the veal instead. Tuscan White Bean Soup makes a perfect starter for this meal (see recipe page 133).

2 tbsp	grated Parmesan cheese
1 ½ tsp	Italian herb seasoning
½ tsp	each salt and pepper
1 lb	veal scallopini or leg cutlets
1 cup	heated low-fat pasta sauce
¼ cup	shredded part-skim mozzarella cheese
2 tbsp	chopped fresh Italian parsley or basil (optional)

—

1. In small bowl, combine cheese, Italian herb seasoning, salt and pepper. Sprinkle on both sides of veal scallopini.

2. Place veal on greased grill over high heat. Close lid and grill, turning once, for about 5 minutes or until no longer pink inside. Place in shallow dish; pour sauce over top and sprinkle with mozzarella and parsley (if using).

Makes 4 servings.

—

Skillet Option: If a grill is unavailable, you can cook the cutlets in a non-stick skillet or grill pan with 2 tsp extra-virgin olive oil.

Vegetarian Option: You can use 1 eggplant, sliced into ½-inch thick slices, instead of the veal. Brush slices with 1 tbsp extra-virgin olive oil then sprinkle with mixture. Grill over medium-high heat for 20 minutes or until tender. Proceed with recipe.

Pork Tenderloin with Grainy Mustard and Chive Crust GREEN-LIGHT

Pork is a very lean meat and is delicious when paired with mustard. Try different kinds such as Dijon or herb-flavoured mustard for variety. Serve this with carrots, broccoli and couscous for a quick but elegant dinner.

1	pork tenderloin, about 12 oz
¼ cup	grainy mustard
1	clove garlic, minced
2 tbsp	chopped fresh chives or green onion
1 tsp	canola oil

—

1. Using sharp knife, trim any excess fat from tenderloin.

2. In small bowl, combine mustard, garlic, chives and oil. Spread evenly over pork tenderloin. Place on small parchment paper– or aluminum foil–lined baking sheet. Roast in 425°F oven for about 18 minutes or until hint of pink remains inside.

3. Place under broiler for 1 minute to brown; turn and repeat with other side. Let stand for 5 minutes. Slice thinly.

Make 3 servings.

—

Helpful Hint: Chop up any leftovers and add to a salad.

Hearty Veal Stew

This is one of my favourite recipes to make on the weekend. Long cooking makes the veal melt in your mouth. You can also try beef or pork in this recipe.

1 ½ lb	lean boneless veal shoulder
2 tbsp	whole wheat flour
2 tsp	Italian herb seasoning
½ tsp	each salt and pepper
2 tbsp	canola oil
2	onions, sliced
4	cloves garlic, minced
1	each stalk celery and carrot, chopped
3 cups	beef stock (low fat, low sodium)
¼ cup	dried porcini mushrooms
¼ cup	tomato paste
1 tbsp	Worcestershire sauce
1	can (540 ml) white kidney beans, drained and rinsed
1 cup	snow peas, halved

—

1. Trim veal of any visible fat. Cut into 1-inch cubes; set aside.

2. In shallow dish or pie plate, combine flour, Italian herb seasoning, salt and pepper. Toss veal with flour mixture.

3. In large shallow pot, heat oil over medium-high heat. Brown veal in batches and remove to plate. Reduce heat to medium and cook onions, garlic, celery, carrot and any remaining flour mixture for 5 minutes or until starting to turn golden. Add stock, mushrooms, tomato paste and Worcestershire sauce. Bring to boil; return veal to pot.

4. Reduce heat; cover and simmer for about 1 hour or until veal is tender. Uncover and add beans and snow peas. Cook for another 15 minutes or until snow peas are tender-crisp.

Makes 6 servings.

—

Veal with Fennel and Mushrooms

GREEN-LIGHT

Veal is a lean and tender cut and is wonderful paired with the aromatic flavour of fennel. Fennel, also called anise, can be found in the produce section of your grocery store and has a mild licorice flavour.

1 lb	veal scallopini
¾ tsp	salt
½ tsp	pepper
1 tbsp	extra-virgin olive oil
1 lb	mushrooms, sliced
Half	fennel bulb, thinly sliced
2 tsp	dried sage leaves or 2 tbsp chopped fresh sage
½ cup	dry white or Marsala wine
¼ cup	chopped fresh Italian parsley

1. Using meat pounder, pound veal to $\frac{1}{8}$-inch thickness. Sprinkle with ½ tsp of the salt, and the pepper.

2. In large non-stick skillet, heat half of the oil over medium-high heat. Cook veal in batches for 2 minutes per side or until browned. Remove to plate; keep warm.

3. Return skillet to heat and add remaining oil. Cook mushrooms, fennel, sage and remaining salt for 15 minutes or until all liquid is evaporated and mushrooms are beginning to brown. Add wine and boil for 3 minutes. Pour sauce over veal and sprinkle with parsley.

Makes 4 servings.

Veal Piccata Option: Instead of using wine, use ¼ cup lemon juice and ½ tsp grated lemon rind and boil for 1 minute. Add 1 tbsp chopped capers.

Chunky Lamb and Bean Stew   YELLOW-LIGHT

The beans in this dish provide a creamy sauce for the lamb. If you haven't tried this classic combination, it could become a new favourite of your family's.

1 ½ lb	lean boneless lamb
1 tbsp	canola oil
2	onions, chopped
2	cloves garlic, minced
1 tbsp	chopped fresh thyme leaves or 1 tsp dried
2 tsp	chopped fresh rosemary or ½ tsp dried
½ tsp	red pepper flakes
½ tsp	each salt and pepper
3 cups	beef stock (low fat, low sodium)
1	bay leaf
1	can (540 ml) white kidney beans, drained and rinsed
1	tomato, chopped
¼ cup	chopped fresh Italian parsley

—

1. Cut lamb into ½-inch cubes. In large shallow saucepan, heat oil over medium-high heat and brown lamb. Remove to plate. Reduce heat to medium and add onions, garlic, thyme, rosemary, red pepper flakes, salt and pepper. Cook for about 5 minutes or until softened.

2. Add beef stock, bay leaf and browned lamb to onion mixture. Bring to boil; cover and reduce heat and simmer for 1 hour.

3. Meanwhile, using potato masher, mash beans coarsely. Add beans, tomato and parsley to lamb; cover and continue cooking for about 30 minutes or until lamb is very tender and sauce is thickened. Remove bay leaf.

Makes 4 servings.

—

Pork Tenderloin
with Apple Compote
GREEN-LIGHT

Serve this comforting dish with Brussels sprouts, sliced carrots and some boiled new potatoes tossed in lemon juice and parsley.

1 tbsp	Dijon mustard
½ tsp	dried sage leaves
¼ tsp	dried thyme leaves
Pinch	each salt and pepper
1	pork tenderloin, about 12 oz
1 tbsp	canola oil

Apple Compote:

1 tsp	canola oil
2	small apples, cored and diced
1	onion, finely chopped
¼ tsp	dried thyme leaves
Pinch	each salt and pepper
¼ cup	currants
2 tbsp	apple juice

1. In small bowl, stir together mustard, sage, thyme, salt and pepper. Rub mixture all over tenderloin.

2. In ovenproof non-stick skillet, heat oil over medium-high heat. Brown tenderloin on one side, turn over and place skillet in 400°F oven for about 20 minutes or until pork has only a hint of pink inside. Let stand for 5 minutes before slicing.

3. Apple Compote: Meanwhile, in another non-stick skillet, heat oil over medium-high heat. Cook apples, onion, thyme, salt and pepper for 5 minutes or until light golden. Add currants and apple juice; cook for 1 minute or until apples are tender-crisp. Slice tenderloin and serve with Apple Compote.

Makes 3 servings.

Pork Amandine

This meal can be ready faster than it takes to set the table! Serve with a big helping of steamed green beans or asparagus.

4	fast-fry boneless pork loin chops
1	clove garlic, minced
¼ tsp	dried thyme leaves
Pinch	each salt and pepper
1 tsp	canola oil
¼ cup	dry white wine
¼ cup	chicken stock
½ tsp	cornstarch
2 tbsp	sliced almonds, toasted
1 tbsp	chopped fresh Italian parsley

—

1. Sprinkle pork chops with garlic, thyme, salt and pepper. In large non-stick skillet, heat oil over medium-high heat. Cook chops, turning once, for 5 minutes or until browned; remove to plate.

2. Return skillet to heat and add wine and stock. Bring to boil and cook for 1 minute. Whisk cornstarch with 2 tsp of water and pour into wine mixture. Cook, stirring, for 30 seconds. Return pork chops to pan, turning to coat. Sprinkle with almonds and parsley.

Makes 2 servings.

—

Chicken Stock Option: If you don't want to use wine in this recipe, simply use the same amount of chicken stock. Stir in 1 tsp lemon juice to add some tang to the sauce.

Helpful Hint: If fast-fry boneless pork loin chops are unavailable, you can use boneless pork loin chops that have been pounded to ⅛-inch thickness.

Pesto Pork Chops   YELLOW-LIGHT

This is a quick and easy dinner to put on the table during a busy work week.

4	boneless pork loin chops
¼ cup	pesto
¼ tsp	each salt and pepper
1 tsp	canola oil
1	onion, sliced
1	red pepper, thinly sliced
½ tsp	dried oregano
⅓ cup	chicken stock

—

1. In non-stick skillet, brown pork chops on both sides over medium-high heat. Remove to plate; spread chops with pesto and sprinkle with half each of the salt and pepper; set aside.

2. To same skillet, add oil, onion, red pepper, oregano, and remaining salt and pepper. Cook, stirring, over medium-high heat for about 4 minutes or until golden. Add stock and pork chops, pesto side up. Cover and continue cooking for about 5 minutes or until pork chops have just a hint of pink inside.

Makes 4 servings.

—

Green-Light Chicken Option: You can use 4 boneless skinless chicken breasts or 8 boneless skinless chicken thighs instead of the pork chops.

Pesto Option: Look for sundried tomato pesto in your grocery store and use it in this recipe for a new taste.

Apple Pork Chops

For this dish, choose a cooking apple such as Crispin, Golden Delicious or Northern Spy. Because the sauce is so lovely, be sure to serve these chops with basmati rice.

4	boneless pork loin chops
½ tsp	salt
Pinch	pepper
1 tsp	canola oil
2	apples, cored and sliced
1	large onion, sliced
1 cup	water
2 tbsp	raisins
1	bay leaf
1 ½ tsp	blackstrap molasses
1 ½ tsp	cider vinegar
¼ tsp	dried thyme leaves
2 tsp	cornstarch

1. Trim all fat from pork chops. Sprinkle chops with half of the salt and pepper.

2. In large non-stick skillet, heat oil over medium-high heat and brown chops on both sides. Spread chops with apples and onion. Pour in all but 2 tbsp of the water. Sprinkle with raisins, bay leaf, molasses, vinegar, thyme and remaining salt. Bring to boil. Cover, reduce heat, and simmer for about 45 minutes or until pork is tender.

3. Remove lid and whisk together cornstarch and reserved water. Pour into skillet and cook, stirring, for about 1 minute or until sauce is slightly thickened. Remove bay leaf.

Makes 4 servings.

Apricot-Sage
Stuffed Pork Chops

These pork chops are wonderful entertaining fare. Serve with green beans and carrots tossed with a touch of extra-virgin olive oil and garlic.

4	thick, boneless pork loin chops
Pinch	each salt and pepper
2 tsp	canola oil

Stuffing:

1 tsp	canola oil
1	small onion, minced
2	cloves garlic, minced
2 tbsp	chopped fresh sage leaves or 2 tsp dried
Half	red bell pepper, diced
1 cup	fresh whole wheat bread crumbs
1/4 cup	diced dried apricots
1/4 cup	chopped fresh Italian parsley
1/3 cup	liquid egg
1/4 tsp	each salt and pepper

—

1. Stuffing: In non-stick skillet, heat oil over medium heat. Cook onion, garlic, sage and red pepper for 6 minutes or until softened. Stir in bread crumbs, apricots and parsley; remove from heat. Stir in liquid egg, salt and pepper until well combined. Set aside.

2. Butterfly pork chops almost all the way through, leaving one long side attached, open like a book. Divide stuffing among chops and fold other side over stuffing. Sprinkle with salt and pepper.

3. In non-stick skillet, heat oil over medium-high heat. Brown pork chops on both sides. Place on parchment paper– or aluminum foil–lined baking sheet and roast in 425°F oven for about 20 minutes or until just a hint of pink remains in centre of pork.

Makes 4 servings.

—

Green-Light Chicken Option: You can use 4 boneless skinless chicken breasts instead of the pork chops.

Artichoke and Pork Stew   YELLOW-LIGHT

Canned artichokes need a good rinse before using to remove the brine flavour. Serve with rice and mesclun greens tossed with balsamic vinegar and pepper.

1 ½ lb	boneless pork loin chops
2 tbsp	whole wheat flour
1 tsp	ground cumin
¼ tsp	each turmeric and ground coriander
¼ tsp	salt
Pinch	each cinnamon and cloves
2 tbsp	canola oil (approx)
1 cup	chicken stock (low fat, low sodium) or water
2	onions, chopped
2	cloves garlic, minced
1	carrot, chopped
1	green bell pepper, chopped
1	can (796 ml) diced tomatoes
1	can (398 ml) artichoke hearts, drained and rinsed and quartered
1 cup	frozen peas

—

1. Cut pork chops into ½-inch-thick strips; set aside. In shallow dish or pie plate, combine flour, cumin, turmeric, coriander, salt, cinnamon and cloves; toss pork strips with flour mixture.

2. In large shallow pot, heat 1 tbsp of the oil over medium-high heat; brown pork in batches, adding more oil if necessary. Remove to plate. Add stock to pot and scrape up brown bits, stirring constantly. Add onion, garlic, carrot and pepper; cook for 5 minutes. Add tomatoes and bring to boil. Return meat and juices to pan; reduce heat, cover and simmer for about 1 hour or until pork is tender.

3. Add artichokes and peas and cook, uncovered, for 15 minutes or until slightly thickened.

Makes 6 servings.

—

Snacks

Dried Chickpeas

This is an addictive snack with all the crunch and saltiness of chips and pretzels but without the fat!

2	cans (540 ml each) chickpeas, drained and rinsed
2 tbsp	extra-virgin olive oil or canola oil
½ tsp	salt
Pinch	cayenne

—

1. In large bowl, toss chickpeas with oil, salt and cayenne. Spread onto large baking sheet in a single layer.

2. Bake in 400°F oven, shaking pan a couple of times during cooking, for about 45 minutes, or until golden. Let cool completely.

   Makes about 3 cups.

—

Helpful Hint: You can add more salt or other spices if you would like to change the flavour of the chickpeas.

Sage and Tomato White Bean Dip

GREEN-LIGHT

I like to serve this at parties with vegetables and whole wheat pita crisps. It's also great smeared over a turkey sandwich.

2 tbsp	chopped sundried tomatoes
¼ cup	boiling water
1	can (540 ml) white kidney beans, drained and rinsed
2 tbsp	extra-virgin olive oil
½ tsp	salt
Pinch	pepper
1 tbsp	chopped fresh sage leaves or ½ tsp dried
1	small clove garlic, minced

—

1. Place tomatoes in boiling water; let stand for 10 minutes. Drain and reserve water.

2. In food processor, purée together beans, tomatoes, oil, salt and pepper and 2 tbsp of the reserved water until smooth. Pulse in sage and garlic.

Makes 1 ½ cups.

—

Storage: Keep in airtight container, refrigerated, for up to 2 weeks.

Fresh Fruit Bowl   GREEN-LIGHT

Keep this in the fridge and scoop up bowlfuls for an afternoon snack or after-dinner pick-me-up.

2	oranges
2	kiwis, peeled and sliced
2	nectarines, pitted and sliced
1	star fruit, sliced (optional)
1 cup	halved strawberries
1 cup	red or green seedless grapes
1 cup	blueberries or raspberries
1 tbsp	sugar substitute
2 tsp	lemon juice
Pinch	ground ginger

—

1. Using serrated knife, cut both ends off oranges. Using sawing motion, cut peel and pith off oranges. Over a large bowl, cut orange sections between membranes. Into another small bowl, squeeze any juice from reserved membranes; set aside.

2. Add kiwis, nectarines, star fruit (if using), strawberries, grapes and blueberries to oranges. Toss to combine.

3. Add sugar substitute, lemon juice and ginger to reserved orange juice. Pour over fruit.

Makes 4 cups, enough for 4 servings.

—

Storage: Cover and refrigerate for up to 2 days.

Serving Option: You can sprinkle the fruit with sliced almonds and serve with a dollop of yogurt, if desired.

Roasted Red Pepper Hummus   GREEN-LIGHT

Serve this as a dip with raw veggies or as a spread for sandwiches or hamburgers. You could also enjoy it on its own in half a whole wheat pita with tomatoes and cucumber slices.

1	can (540 ml) chickpeas, drained and rinsed
½ cup	chopped roasted red peppers
¼ cup	tahini
½ tsp	ground cumin
½ tsp	salt
2 tbsp	extra-virgin olive oil
2 tbsp	water
1 tbsp	lemon juice
1	small clove garlic, minced

—

1. In food processor, pulse together chickpeas, peppers, tahini, cumin and salt. With food processor running, add oil and water until very smooth. Pulse in lemon juice and garlic.

Makes about 1 ½ cups.

—

Sundried Tomato Version: Omit roasted red peppers. Use ¼ cup chopped sundried tomatoes that have been rehydrated in hot water and drained.

Roasted Vegetable Hummus: Omit roasted red peppers. Use ½ cup chopped roasted vegetables.

Storage: Keep in airtight container, refrigerated, for up to 2 weeks.

Helpful Hint: Tahini is a sesame seed paste that you can find in most grocery stores. You can also find it in health and bulk food stores. It adds a great nutty flavour to the hummus.

Baked Apple

I love this recipe because it's so quick and easy and you can double or triple it as need be. Baked apples make a delicious sweet snack— and they're also very healthy. You could even have this for breakfast.

1	apple
3 tbsp	Muesli (see recipe page 115)
1 tbsp	non-hydrogenated soft margarine
1 tbsp	raisins
2 tsp	sugar substitute
Pinch	cinnamon or nutmeg

—

1. Using an apple corer or melon baller, remove core from apple. Place apple on small plate or bowl.

2. Combine Muesli, margarine, raisins and sugar substitute and stuff into centre of apple. Any excess should be pressed on top of apple. Sprinkle with cinnamon. Cover loosely with plastic wrap. Microwave on High for about 3 minutes or until apple is tender when pierced with knife.

Makes 1 serving.

—

Helpful Hint: Microwave cooking times will vary depending on the wattage of your microwave. You can check the apple halfway through and determine how much longer it needs to bake.

Pear Option: Omit the apple and use a firm, ripe Bartlett or Bosc pear. It will take less time to cook the pear.

Whole Wheat Scones GREEN-LIGHT

Have these scones with a hot cup of tea in the afternoon. The sweet fruit version makes a wonderful breakfast treat when spread with a little sugar-free fruit spread.

1 ½ cups	whole wheat flour
½ cup	oat bran
3	green onions, chopped
3 tbsp	flax or sunflower seeds
2 tsp	baking powder
2 tsp	sugar substitute
½ tsp	salt
¼ tsp	nutmeg
¼ cup	non-hydrogenated soft margarine
⅔ cup	skim milk
2 tbsp	liquid egg

—

1. In large bowl, combine flour, oat bran, onions, flax seeds, baking powder, sugar substitute, salt and nutmeg. Using your fingers, rub margarine into flour mixture to combine. Add milk and toss with fork to make soft dough.

2. Place dough onto floured surface and knead gently about 5 times. Pat dough out to ½-inch thickness. Cut dough into 8 squares, or use cookie or biscuit cutter to cut scones. Place on baking sheet and brush tops with liquid egg. Bake in 425°F oven for about 12 minutes or until golden on bottom.

Makes 8 scones.

—

Sweet Fruit Option: Omit green onions and flax seeds. Increase sugar substitute to 2 tbsp and add ½ cup chopped dried apricots, raisins or dried cranberries.

Orange Bran Muffins   YELLOW-LIGHT

Ruth enjoys making these muffins for Rick and many of their friends. Though the recipe calls for a whole orange, the sugar substitute removes the bitterness of the rind. Use a navel orange, which has no seeds and is very juicy.

1	orange, unpeeled
¾ cup	skim milk
½ cup	orange juice
¼ cup	non-hydrogenated soft margarine
1	egg
1 tsp	vanilla
2 cups	whole wheat flour
½ cup	wheat bran
¼ cup	sugar substitute
1 tsp	baking powder
1 tsp	baking soda
1 tsp	cinnamon
Pinch	salt

—

1. Cut orange into 8 wedges. Place in food processor bowl and pulse until finely chopped or almost puréed. Add milk, orange juice, margarine, egg and vanilla; purée until combined.

2. In large bowl, combine flour, bran, sugar substitute, baking powder, baking soda, cinnamon and salt. Pour orange mixture over flour mixture and stir until just combined. Divide batter among 12 lined or greased muffin cups. Bake in 400°F oven for about 20 minutes or until golden and firm to the touch.

Makes 12 muffins.

—

Storage: These muffins can be kept at room temperature for about 2 days or frozen for up to 1 month.

Cranberry Cinnamon Bran Muffins

My aunt Carmen is a nurse and likes to make big batches of these muffins to bring to her co-workers on the nightshift. They are very nutritious, with a high fibre content, and have a great cinnamon flavour.

1 cup	wheat bran
½ cup	All-Bran or 100% Bran cereal
¼ tsp	salt
½ cup	boiling water
1 cup	skim milk
1 cup	dried cranberries
⅓ cup	sugar substitute
1	egg
¼ cup	canola oil
1 ¼ cups	whole wheat flour
1 ¼ tsp	baking soda
1 tsp	cinnamon

—

1. In bowl, combine bran, cereal and salt. Pour boiling water over and stir to combine. Stir in milk and cranberries and set aside.

2. In another bowl, whisk together sugar substitute, egg and oil. Stir into bran mixture.

3. In large bowl, stir together flour, baking soda and cinnamon. Pour bran mixture over flour mixture and stir until just combined. Divide batter among 12 lined or greased muffin cups. Bake in 375°F oven for about 20 minutes or until tester inserted in centre comes out clean.

Makes 12 muffins.

—

Storage: These muffins can be kept at room temperature for about 2 days or frozen for up to 1 month. Wrap each muffin individually before freezing to help prevent freezer burn. Then place them in a resealable plastic bag or airtight container.

Lemon Blueberry Muffins   YELLOW-LIGHT

Lemon and blueberries have a natural affinity for each other. You can wrap these muffins individually in plastic wrap and store them in large resealable plastic bags in the freezer. When you feel like having one, let it come to room temperature or pop it in the microwave for that fresh-out-of-the-oven taste.

1 ½ cups	whole wheat flour
½ cup	wheat bran
½ cup	sugar substitute
1 tbsp	baking powder
½ tsp	salt
1 cup	skim milk
1	egg
¼ cup	non-hydrogenated soft margarine, melted, or canola oil
1 tbsp	grated lemon rind
1 cup	fresh or frozen blueberries

—

1. In large bowl, combine flour, bran, sugar substitute, baking powder and salt. In small bowl, whisk together milk, egg, margarine and lemon rind. Pour milk mixture over flour mixture and stir just until combined. Stir in blueberries.

2. Divide batter among 9 lined or greased muffin cups. Fill remaining empty muffin cups in pan with a bit of water to prevent burning. Bake in 375°F oven for about 20 minutes or until golden and firm to the touch.

Makes 9 muffins.

—

Helpful Hint: If using frozen blueberries, do not thaw. Add them directly into the batter.

Storage: These muffins can be kept at room temperature for about 2 days or frozen for up to 3 weeks.

Apple Raisin Bread   YELLOW-LIGHT

*A slice of this bread makes a delicious afternoon snack. You can
also toast it and top it with a little margarine. Keep this bread
wrapped in plastic wrap and aluminum foil to lengthen its storage.
It freezes well for up to one month.*

1 ¼ cups	whole wheat flour
½ cup	wheat bran
½ cup	sugar substitute
2 tsp	cinnamon
1 tsp	baking powder
½ tsp	baking soda
¼ tsp	nutmeg
¼ tsp	salt
2	apples, cored and diced
⅓ cup	raisins
⅓ cup	chopped pecans or almonds (optional)
1 cup	buttermilk
⅓ cup	liquid egg
¼ cup	canola oil
2 tbsp	brown sugar substitute (optional)

—

1. In large bowl, combine flour, bran, sugar substitute, cinnamon,
   baking powder, baking soda, nutmeg and salt. Toss in apples,
   raisins and pecans (if using) to coat with flour.

2. Whisk together buttermilk, liquid egg and oil. Pour over flour
   mixture and stir until just combined. Pour batter into 9- x 5-inch
   greased loaf pan. Sprinkle top with brown sugar substitute (if
   using). Bake in 350 F oven for about 45 minutes or until golden
   and tester inserted in centre comes out clean. Let cool on rack.

Makes 1 loaf, or 12 slices.

—

Helpful Hint: You don't have buttermilk in your refrigerator? No problem, you can make soured milk, which is a perfect substitute. Add 1 tbsp lemon juice or white vinegar to 1 cup skim milk. Let stand for a couple of minutes. Stir, and presto—you have soured milk.

Desserts

Poached Pears GREEN-LIGHT

Poaching pears in fruit juice adds to their sweetness and gives them a richer flavour. Serve with a dollop of Yogurt Cheese (recipe page 114) or low-fat, no-added-sugar ice cream.

2 cups	pear juice
4	black peppercorns
2	whole cloves
1	cinnamon stick
2	pears, cored and quartered

—

1. In saucepan, bring juice, peppercorns, cloves and cinnamon stick to boil. Reduce heat to simmer and add pears. Simmer for about 10 minutes or until pears are tender when pierced with knife. Remove to bowl.

2. Bring juice mixture to boil again. Boil for 3 minutes. Strain over pears.

Makes 2 servings.

—

Helpful Hint: Look for ripe pears by picking them up and pressing gently on their skin. If a pear yields slightly and smells fresh and ripe, then that's the one you want to bring home.

Basmati Rice Pudding

Here is quintessential comfort food to warm the heart and soul. Try serving this with other favourite fruits such as strawberries or plums.

3 cups	skim milk
½ cup	basmati rice
¼ cup	sugar substitute
1 tsp	vanilla
¼ tsp	ground cardamom or cinnamon
2	peaches or nectarines, peeled and sliced thinly

—

1. In heavy saucepan, bring milk and rice to boil over medium heat. Reduce heat to low; stir and cover and cook for about 30 minutes or until most of the milk is absorbed. Stir in sugar substitute, vanilla and cardamom.

2. Spoon into 4 custard cups and top with sliced peaches.

Makes 4 servings.

—

Berry Crumble

This is one of Ruth's favourite green-light desserts. Though it's best made with fresh berries during the summer, it's also lovely with frozen fruit.

5 cups	fresh or frozen berries, such as raspberries, black- berries, blueberries and sliced strawberries
1	large apple, cored and chopped
2 tbsp	whole wheat flour
2 tbsp	sugar substitute
½ tsp	cinnamon

Topping:

1 cup	large-flake oats
½ cup	chopped pecans or walnuts
¼ cup	brown sugar substitute
¼ cup	non-hydrogenated soft margarine, melted
1 tsp	cinnamon

—

1. In 8-inch square baking dish, combine berries and apple. In bowl, combine flour, sugar substitute and cinnamon. Sprinkle over fruit and toss gently.

2. Topping: In bowl, combine oats, pecans, brown sugar substitute, margarine and cinnamon. Sprinkle over fruit mixture. Bake in 350°F oven for about 30 minutes or until fruit is tender and top is golden.

Makes 6 servings.

—

Microwave Option: Prepare as above and microwave on High for about 6 minutes or until fruit is tender. The top won't get golden or crisp in the microwave.

Glazed Apple Tart

This tart is worthy enough to serve to company and is especially pretty made with red-skinned apples.

1 cup	whole almonds
½ cup	dried whole wheat cracker or bread crumbs
1 tsp	cinnamon
2	egg whites, lightly beaten
½ cup	unsweetened applesauce
1	egg
2 tbsp	sugar substitute
¼ tsp	almond extract
2	apples, cored
2 tbsp	unsweetened apricot or peach jam

—

1. Place almonds on baking sheet and toast in 350°F oven for about 10 minutes or until fragrant. Let cool.

2. In food processor, grind almonds finely; place in bowl. Add bread crumbs and ½ tsp of the cinnamon; toss to combine. Add egg whites and stir to combine. Press mixture into bottom and up sides of 8-inch pie plate. Bake in 350°F oven for about 10 minutes or until firm. Let cool.

3. In bowl, whisk together applesauce, egg, sugar substitute, remaining cinnamon and almond extract. Spread over bottom of crust.

4. Cut apples in half and cut thin half-moon-shaped slices. Place in concentric circles over applesauce mixture. Bake in 400°F oven for about 15 minutes or until apples are tender when pierced with knife. Brush top with jam. Let cool on rack.

Makes 6 servings.

—

Baked Chocolate Mousse   GREEN-LIGHT

Seemingly sinful, this mousse is dense and rich. Make it on the weekend to enjoy throughout the week.

1 cup	skim milk
3 oz	unsweetened chocolate, chopped
½ cup	liquid egg
1 cup	sugar substitute
2 tsp	vanilla

—

1. In saucepan, heat milk over medium heat until steaming. Whisk in chocolate until melted.

2. In bowl, whisk together liquid egg, sugar substitute and vanilla. Gradually whisk milk mixture into egg mixture until combined. Pour into 4 custard cups or ramekins. Place cups into 8-inch baking dish. Fill baking dish with boiling water halfway up around custard cups.

3. Bake in 325°F oven for about 25 minutes or until knife inserted in centre comes out creamy.

Makes 4 servings.

—

Helpful Hint: Let cool completely before refrigerating so no water droplets will form on the surface.

Storage: Cover with plastic wrap and refrigerate for up to 1 week.

Almond Bran Haystacks

GREEN-LIGHT

These cookies are best the day they are baked. After that they tend to lose their crispness, though they still taste yummy. Enjoy them with a cup of decaf coffee or skim milk.

2	egg whites
¼ tsp	cream of tartar
⅓ cup	sugar substitute
1 ¼ cups	All-Bran or 100% Bran cereal
½ cup	chopped almonds, toasted
1 tbsp	vanilla
¼ tsp	almond extract

—

1. In large bowl, beat egg whites and cream of tartar until soft peaks form. Gradually add sugar substitute and beat until stiff peaks form. Fold in cereal, almonds, vanilla and almond extract until combined.

2. Drop batter by tablespoonfuls onto parchment paper–lined baking sheet. Bake in 325°F oven for about 15 minutes or until lightly browned and firm to the touch. Let cool completely.

Makes about 18 cookies.

—

Storage: Keep in airtight container for up to 5 days. These do not freeze well.

Apple Pie Cookies

These cookies combine all the flavours of traditional apple pie and have a texture similar to that of a soft granola bar. A great snack!

1 cup	large-flake oatmeal
3/4 cup	whole wheat flour
1 tsp	cinnamon
1/2 tsp	baking powder
Pinch	each nutmeg and salt
3/4 cup	unsweetened applesauce
1/3 cup	sugar substitute
1/3 cup	liquid egg
2 tsp	vanilla
1	apple, cored and finely diced

—

1. In large bowl, combine oatmeal, flour, cinnamon, baking powder, nutmeg and salt. In another bowl, whisk together applesauce, sugar substitute, liquid egg and vanilla. Pour over oatmeal mixture and stir to combine. Add apple and stir to distribute evenly.

2. Drop by heaping tablespoonfuls onto parchment paper–lined baking sheet. Bake in 275°F oven for about 25 minutes or until firm and lightly golden. Let cool completely.

Makes about 18 cookies.

—

Storage: Keep in airtight container for up to 3 days or freeze for up to 2 weeks.

Pecan Brownies

Brownies, you ask? That's right. These are packed with fibre and are absolutely scrumptious, so get baking!

1	can (540 ml) white or red kidney or black beans, drained and rinsed
½ cup	skim milk
⅓ cup	liquid egg
¼ cup	soft non-hydrogenated margarine, melted
1 tbsp	vanilla
¾ cup	sugar substitute
½ cup	whole wheat flour
½ cup	unsweetened cocoa powder
1 tsp	baking powder
Pinch	salt
½ cup	chopped toasted pecans

—

1. In food processor, purée beans until coarse. Add in milk, liquid egg, margarine and vanilla and purée until smooth, scraping down sides a few times. Set aside.

2. In large bowl, combine sugar substitute, flour, cocoa, baking powder and salt. Pour bean mixture over flour mixture. Stir to combine. Scrape batter into parchment paper–lined 8-inch square baking pan, smoothing top. Sprinkle with pecans.

3. Bake in 350°F oven for about 18 minutes or until cake tester inserted in centre comes out clean. Let cool on rack.

Makes 16 brownies.

—

Storage: Cover these brownies with plastic wrap or store them in an airtight container for up to 4 days. They can also be frozen for up to 2 weeks.

Appendix I

Green-Light Glossary

The following is a summary of the most popular green-light foods.

Almonds

This is the perfect nut in that it has the highest monounsaturated fat (good fat) content of any nut, and recent research indicates that almonds can significantly lower LDL, or bad, cholesterol. They are also excellent sources of Vitamin E, fibre and protein. They provide a great boost to the beneficial fat content of your meals, especially at breakfast or in salads and desserts. Because all nuts are high in calories, use them in moderation.

Apples

A real staple. Eat them fresh for a snack or dessert. Unsweetened applesauce goes well with cereals, or with cottage cheese as a snack.

Barley

An excellent supplement to soups.

Beans

If there's one food you can never get enough of, it's beans, or legumes. This perfect green-light food is high in protein and fibre and can supplement nearly every meal. Make bean salads or just add beans to any salad. Add them to soups, use them to replace some of the meat in casseroles or put them in a meat loaf. You can serve them as a side vegetable or as an alternative to potatoes, rice or pasta.

A wide range of canned and frozen beans is available. Exercise some caution with baked beans, as the sauce can be high-fat and high-calorie. Check labels for low-fat, low-sugar versions and watch the size of your serving.

Beans have a well-deserved reputation for creating "wind," so be patient until your body adapts—as it will—to your increased consumption.

Bread

Most breads are red-light except for 100% stone-ground whole wheat or coarse whole grain breads that have around 2½ to 3 grams of fibre per slice (not serving). Check labels carefully as the bread industry likes to confuse the unwary. The wording to look for on packages is "100% stone-ground." Most bread is made from flour that is ground by steel rollers, which strip away the bran coating, leaving a very fine powder ideal for producing light, fluffy breads and pastries. Conversely, stone-ground flour is coarser and retains more of its bran coating, so it is digested more slowly in your stomach. Even with bread made from whole grains, you have to watch your quantity. Have only one slice per meal.

Cereals

Use only large-flake porridge oats, oat bran or other high-fibre cold cereals that have ten grams of fibre or more per serving. Though these cereals are not much fun in themselves, you can liven them up with fruit or fruit-flavoured fat- and sugar-free yogurt or even sugar-reduced fruit spreads. If you wish to sweeten your cereal, use a sweetener, not sugar.

Cottage cheese

One percent or fat-free cottage cheese is an excellent low-fat, high-protein food. Add fruit to it for a snack or add it to salads.

Eggs

As long as you stick to liquid low-cholesterol and low-fat eggs such as Break Free or Omega Pro, you needn't limit your intake of them. In fact, you should make them a regular part of your diet. In Phase II, if you'd really rather use whole eggs, buy the omega-3 kind, which are a little lower in cholesterol than regular eggs. The omega-3 content is beneficial for heart health.

Fish/Shellfish

These are ideal green-light foods, low in fat and cholesterol and a good source of protein. Some coldwater fish such as salmon are also rich in omega-3. Never eat battered or breaded fish.

Food bars

Most food or nutrition bars are dietary disasters, high in carbohydrates and calories but low in protein. These bars are simply quick sugar fixes. There are a few, such as Balance and Power Protein bars, that have a more equitable distribution of carbohydrates, proteins and fats. Look for 20 to 30 grams of carbohydrates, 12 to 15 grams of protein and 5 grams of fat. This comes to about 220 calories per bar. A real bargain is the Shoppers Drug Mart brand of food bars. Keep them at home and at work for a convenient snack— remember that the serving size is half of one bar. In an emergency, it's okay to have one bar plus an apple and a glass of skim milk for lunch if you can't get away for a proper break. But try not to make a habit of it.

Grapefruit

One of the top-rated green-light foods. Eat grapefruit as often as you like.

Hamburgers

These are acceptable only if they have been made with extra-lean ground beef that has 10 percent or less fat. You can add some oat bran to the meat to provide more fibre and less fat. Alternatively, you could use ground turkey or chicken. And there are some soy substitutes for meat that taste remarkably good and are worth checking out. Keep the serving size at four ounces and eat open-faced with only half of a whole wheat bun.

Meat

The best green-light meats are skinless chicken and turkey, fully trimmed beef, veal, deli cuts of lean ham, and back bacon. The beef cuts to choose are round, top sirloin or tenderloin.

Milk

Use skim only. If you have trouble adjusting to it, then use 1% and slowly wean yourself off it. The fat you're giving up is saturated. Milk is a terrific snack or meal supplement. I drink two glasses of skim milk a day, at breakfast and lunch.

Nuts

Nuts are a principal source of "good" fat, which is essential for your health. Almonds are your best choice. Add them to cereals, salads and desserts. Because they are calorie dense, they must be used in moderation.

Oat bran

You can use this excellent high-fibre food in baking as a partial replacement for flour, or you can make it into a hot cereal.

Oatmeal

If you haven't had oatmeal since you were a kid, now's the time to revisit it. Large-flake, or old-fashioned, oatmeal is the breakfast of choice, because not only is it green-light, but it also lowers cholesterol. The instant and quick cooking (one-minute) versions are not recommended because they have a far higher G.I. content due to the extra processing of the oats. I like oatmeal so much, I often have it as a snack with unsweetened applesauce and sweetener (I use ⅓ cup oats).

Oranges

Fresh oranges are excellent as snacks, at breakfast and added to cereals. A glass of orange juice has 2½ times as many calories as a whole orange, so avoid the juice and stick with the real thing.

Pasta

Most pastas are acceptable if you do not overcook them (pasta should be al dente, with some firmness to the bite) and if you limit the serving size to a quarter of your plate. Never use pasta as the basis of a meal—it is a side dish only.

Peaches, pears and plums

These fruits are terrific snacks, desserts or additions to breakfast cereal. Buy them fresh, or canned in water or juice (drain the juice).

Potatoes

Only boiled new potatoes are acceptable on the G.I. Diet. They have a low starch content, unlike the larger, more mature potatoes, which are very red-light. Still, limit your quantity to two or three per serving.

Rice

Various types of rice have different G.I. ratings, and most of them are red-light. The best kinds are basmati and long grain, and brown is better than white. Don't overcook rice so that it starts to clump together. The more it's cooked, the more glutinous and red-light it becomes.

Soups
Canned soups have a higher G.I. rating than homemade ones because of the high temperature at which commercial varieties are processed. I have included some brands of canned soup in the green-light category because these are the best alternative available. Homemade soups are even more green-light.

Sour cream
One percent or non-fat sour cream with a little sweetener stirred in is an ideal alternative to whipped cream as a dessert topping. You can also mix fruit or low-sugar fruit spread into it for a creamy dessert.

Soy
Soy protein powder is a simple way to boost the protein level of any meal. It's particularly useful at breakfast for sprinkling over cereal. Look for the kind that has a 90 percent protein content. It's sometimes labelled "isolated soy protein powder." Unflavoured low- or non-fat soy milk is a perfect green-light beverage.

Sweeteners (Sugar Substitutes)
There has been a tremendous amount of misinformation circulating about artificial sweeteners—all of which has been proven groundless. The sugar industry rightly saw these new products as a threat and has done its best to bad-mouth

them. You can find an excellent medical overview of sugar substitutes in the U.S. Food and Drug Administration Consumer Magazine at www.fda.gov.

Use Splenda, Equal, Sweet'n Low and Sugar Twin to replace sugar in your diet. If you are allergic to sweeteners, then fructose is a better alternative to sugar. The herbal sweetener stevia, which can be found in health food stores, is acceptable if used in moderation since no long-term studies on its usage are available.

Tofu

Though not flavourful in itself, tofu can be spiced up in a variety of ways and is an excellent low-fat source of protein. Use it to boost or replace meat and seafood in stir-fries, burgers and salads.

Yogurt

Non-fat, fruit-flavoured yogurt sweetened with aspartame is a great green-light product and has one of the lowest G.I.s of all foods. It makes an ideal snack or a flavourful addition to breakfast cereal or fruit for dessert. I always keep our refrigerator well stocked with a variety of flavours. In fact, my shopping cart is so full of yogurt containers that fellow shoppers frequently stop me to ask if they are on special!

Yogurt cheese

A wonderful substitute for sour cream in desserts or in main dishes like chili. Emily has provided a recipe for this green-light staple on page 114.

Note: Additional updates can be found at **www.gidiet.com.**

Appendix II

Green-Light Pantry Guide

PANTRY	FRIDGE	FREEZER
BAKING/COOKING	**DAIRY**	**DAIRY**
Baking powder/soda	Buttermilk	Ice cream (low fat and no added sugar)
Cocoa	Cottage cheese (1%)	
Dried apricots	Fruit yogurt (fat- and sugar-free)	
Sliced almonds	Milk (skim)	
Wheat bran	Sour cream (fat-free or 1%)	
Whole wheat flour		
BEANS (CANNED)	**FRUIT**	**MEAT/POULTRY/FISH/EGGS**
Baked (low-fat)	Apples	(see Fridge)
Mixed salad beans	Blueberries	

PANTRY	FRIDGE	FREEZER
Soybeans	Blackberries	**SNACKS**
Vegetarian chili	Cherries	Homemade muffins (see recipes pp. 239–243)
	Grapefruit	
BREADS	Grapes	**VEGETABLES/FRUIT**
100% stone-ground whole wheat	Lemons	Mixed berries
	Limes	Mixed peppers
CEREALS	Oranges	Mixed vegetables
All-Bran	Peaches	Peas
Bran Buds	Pears	
Fibre First	Plums	
Kashi Go Lean	Raspberries	
Oatmeal (large flake)	Strawberries	
Red River		
DRINKS	**MEAT/POULTRY/ FISH/EGGS**	
Bottled water	All seafood (no batter or breading)	
Club soda	Chicken breast (skinless)	
Decaffeinated coffee/tea	Ham/turkey/chicken (lean deli)	
Diet soft drinks	Low-cholesterol liquid eggs (Break Free/Omega Pro)	
	Turkey breast (skinless)	
	Veal	

PANTRY	FRIDGE	FREEZER
FATS/OILS	**VEGETABLES**	
Canola oil	Asparagus	
Margarine (no-fat, light)	Beans (green or wax)	
Mayonnaise (no-fat)	Bell peppers	
Olive oil	Broccoli	
Salad dressings (no-fat)	Cabbage	
Vegetable oil sprays	Carrots	
	Cauliflower	
FRUIT (CANNED/BOTTLED)	Celery	
Applesauce (no sugar)	Cucumber	Berries
Mandarin oranges	Eggplant	Mixed fruit
Peaches in juice or water	Lettuce	
Pears in juice or water	Mushrooms	
	Olives	
PASTA	Onion	
Fettuccine	Peppers (hot)	
Spaghetti	Pickles	
Vermicelli	Potatoes (new only)	
	Radishes	
PASTA SAUCES (vegetable-based only)	Snow peas	
Healthy Choice	Spinach	
Too Good To Be True	Tomatoes	
	Zucchini	

PANTRY	FRIDGE	FREEZER
RICE		
Basmati		
Long-grain		
Wild		
SEASONINGS		
Flavoured vinegars/ sauces		
Spices/herbs		
SNACKS		
Food bars (Power/ Balance)		
SOUPS (vegetable- or bean-based only)		
Healthy Choice		
Healthy Request		
Too Good To Be True		
SWEETENERS		
Equal		
Splenda		
Sugar Twin		
Sweet'n Low		

Appendix III

G.I. Diet Shopping List

PANTRY	FRIDGE/FREEZER
BAKING/COOKING	**DAIRY**
Baking powder/soda	Buttermilk
Cocoa	Cottage cheese (1%)
Dried apricots*	Ice cream (low fat, no added sugar)
Sliced almonds	Milk (skim)
Wheat/oat bran	Sour cream (fat-free or 1%)
Whole wheat flour	Yogurt (fat- and sugar-free)
BEANS (CANNED)	
Baked beans (low-fat)	**FRUIT**
Mixed salad beans	Apples
Most varieties	Blackberries
Vegetarian chili	Blueberries
BREAD	Cherries
100% stone-ground whole wheat	Grapefruit
CEREALS	Grapes
All-Bran	Lemons
Bran Buds	Limes
Fibre First	Oranges
Kashi Go Lean	Peaches
Oatmeal (large flake)	Pears
Soy protein powder	Plums
	Raspberries
	Strawberries

DRINKS	MEAT/POULTRY/FISH/EGGS
Bottled water	All seafood (no batter or breading)
Club soda	Chicken breast (skinless)
Coffee/tea	Extra lean ground beef
Diet soft drinks	Ham/turkey/chicken (lean deli)
FATS/OILS	Liquid eggs (Break Free/Omega Pro)
Almonds	Turkey breast (skinless)
Canola oil	Veal
Margarine (no-fat/light)	**VEGETABLES**
Mayonnaise (no-fat)	Asparagus
Olive oil	Beans (green/wax)
Salad dressings (no-fat)	Bell and hot peppers
Vegetable oil spray	Broccoli
FRUIT (CANNED/BOTTLED)	Cabbage
Applesauce (no sugar)	Carrots
Mandarin oranges	Cauliflower
Peaches in juice or water	Celery
Pears in juice or water	Cucumber
PASTA	Eggplant
Capellini	Leeks
Fettuccine	Lettuce
Macaroni	Mushrooms
Penne	Olives
Spaghetti	Onions
Vermicelli	Pickles
PASTA SAUCES	Potatoes (new/small only)
(vegetable-based only)	Snow peas
Healthy Choice	Spinach
Too Good To Be True	Tomatoes
RICE	Zucchini
Basmati/long grain/wild	**SOUPS**
SEASONINGS	Healthy Choice
Flavoured vinegars/sauces	Too Good To Be True
Spices/herbs	**SWEETENERS**
SNACKS	Equal, Splenda, Sweet'n Low,
Food bars (Power/Balance)	Sugar Twin (and other
	sugar substitutes)

Appendix IV

G.I. Diet
Dining Out Tips

BREAKFAST GREEN LIGHT	BREAKFAST RED LIGHT
All-Bran	Cold cereals
Egg Whites—Omelette	Bacon/sausage
Egg Whites—Scrambled	Eggs
Fruit	Muffins
Oatmeal	Pancakes/waffles
Yogurt (low-fat)	

LUNCH GREEN LIGHT	LUNCH RED LIGHT
Meats—deli style ham/ chicken/turkey breast	Bakery products
Pasta—¼ plate maximum	Butter/mayonnaise
Salads—low-fat (dressing on the side)	Cheese
Sandwiches—open-faced/ whole wheat	Fast food
Soups—chunky vegetable-bean	Pasta-based meals
Vegetables	Pizza/bread/bagels
Wraps—½ whole wheat pita, no mayonnaise	Potatoes (replace with double vegetables)

Dinner Green Light	Dinner Red Light
Chicken/turkey (no skin)	Beef/lamb/pork
Fruit	Bread
Pasta—¼ plate	Butter/mayonnaise
Rice (basmati, brown, wild, long grain)—¼ plate	Caesar salad
Salads—low-fat (dressing on the side)	Desserts
Seafood—not breaded or battered	Potatoes (replace with double vegetables)
Soups—chunky vegetable and bean	Soups—cream based
Vegetables	

Snacks Green Light	Snacks Red Light
Almonds	Chips, all types
Food bar—½ (e.g. Balance)	Cookies/Muffins
Fresh fruit	Popcorn, regular
Hazelnuts	
Yogurt—no fat/no sugar	

Portions	
Meat	Palm of hand / Pack of cards
Rice/pasta	Maximum ¼ plate
Vegetables	Minimum ½ plate

Appendix V

The Ten Golden G.I. Diet Rules

1. Eat three meals and three snacks every day. Don't skip meals—particularly breakfast.

2. Stick with green-light products only in Phase I.

3. When it comes to food, quantity is as important as quality. Shrink your usual portions, particularly of meat, pasta and rice.

4. Always ensure that each meal contains the appropriate measure of carbohydrates, protein and fat.

5. Eat at least three times more vegetables and fruit than usual.

6. Drink plenty of fluids, preferably water.

7. Exercise for thirty minutes once a day or fifteen minutes twice a day. Get off the bus three stops early.

8. Find a friend to join you for mutual support.

9. Set realistic goals. Try to lose an average of a pound a week and record your progress to reinforce your sense of achievement.

10. Don't view this as a diet. It's the basis of how you will eat for the rest of your life.

G.I. DIET WEEKLY WEIGHT/WAIST LOG

WEEK	DATE	WEIGHT	WAIST	COMMENTS
1.				
2.				
3.				
4.				
5.				
6.				
7.				
8.				
9.				
10.				
11.				
12.				
13.				
14.				
15.				
16.				
17.				
18.				
19.				
20.				

Index